DO THIS, EAT THAT

An approach to successful fat loss and body re-composition

ANTHONY CAMPO & KRISTINA MARTEMUCCI

ISBN: 1484978420
ISBN-13: 978-1484978429

SPECIAL THANKS TO

Ben Cabot III Photography
Helena Lukas Martemucci Photography

Cover Design by: Lukáš Urbánek

TABLE OF CONTENTS

"In November 2012, at three-hundred and twenty pounds, I began going to Physical Therapy for a hurting back that was limiting my daily living activities. I was overweight and my doctor wanted to start me on medication for high blood pressure and cholesterol. I met Anthony when he began working with me as my Physical Therapist Assistant. He recommended the Do This, Eat That plan to me to improve my body composition, fitness, and health markers. I stand here today less than nine months later at two-hundred and fifty pounds on my fiftieth birthday. The plan was simple and gave me all of the tools I needed to lose over seventy pounds despite a hectic work schedule. I never dreamed I would now be in such good shape at age fifty! I returned to my doctor to get blood work, and both my blood pressure and cholesterol were now at normal levels. My doctor was so amazed that he thought I was on medication. When I informed him that I never started any medication, but rather started a nutrition/fitness plan he immediately inquired as to what the plan was. I replied that it was simple, just Do This, Eat That!"

-Kevin Polhamus, Food Services Manager

"I have struggled with weight loss despite having a regular exercise routine and what I perceived as a healthy nutrition plan. I work with Kristina as my trainer and she introduced me to the "DO THIS, EAT THAT" nutrition/fitness plan in March 2013. It was easy and fun to fit into my busy schedule, e.g. doing a

5 minute walk, wall push-ups or 20 squats while at work. IT WORKS!! I experienced immediate results. Six months later not only have I lost 17 pounds, but I have kept the weight off despite a summer filled with travel, family gatherings and lots of fun. I encourage anyone to give it a try and commit to 4-8 weeks to start and you will see results and feel better."

Pat, Registered Nurse

PREFACE

It is no secret that in today's world, obesity is out of control and increasing at an alarming rate for individuals everywhere. Obesity is related to many medical and orthopedic issues, and recent studies place obesity responsible for almost 30 percent of total healthcare costs. Our passion for helping to resolve this issue, along with health and fitness in general, has led us to reach out to others. Working in both the training and therapy industries, educating individuals on obesity/disease prevention, and health management through fitness and nutrition are topics that we have spent the better part of a decade studying and practicing. Through higher education, sound research, and practical studies, we have been able to apply simple nutritional and exercise science to improve the body composition of hundreds of people. The key was making this breakthrough information available in a way that any individual, regardless of lifestyle or ability, would be able to implement it into their lives. Born from success stories, and the passion to do things right was *Do This, Eat That.* Though this book is cutting edge, it utilizes time tested methods of science to ensure that you will be improving your body composition in the best way possible. All of the information in this book is not new by any means, but this is the first time it has been put all together into one ultimate body re-composition manual.

INTRODUCTION

In the culture we live in today, the overwhelming health-and-fitness philosophy is that all we need to do is eat less and move more, and we will lose weight. While there is some validity to this thought, there is a little more to it than just that. We are exposed to an endless variety of health-and-fitness magazines that have us tinkering around with a game in which many of us keep losing and regaining five pounds. The philosophy of portion control, treating yourself when it isn't called for (or as the magazines call it, "not depriving" yourself,) and moderate-intensity cardio as our primary source of exercise may get us some positive results at the beginning, but will inevitably leave us stuck playing this five-pound weight game. This game simply involves messing around with glycogen (energy) stores and water weight, and is not an efficient way to lose fat or make progress for the long run.

This popular way of thought simply does not work, and the proof is in the numbers. Record amounts of money have been spent on dieting over the past years, yet obesity is at a higher rate today than ever before. Something isn't working. Perhaps this is due to the fact that the motivation behind the magazine companies is not for us to lose weight but rather to keep us playing this five-pound weight-loss/weight-gain game so we keep buying their magazines and jump on the next trendy diet.

This will inevitably put us right back where we started and the game begins again.

In order to ensure that you lose mostly fat and not muscle, and turn your body into a long-term fat-burning machine, you must learn to eat the way your body was meant to. This is a simple plan that will teach you to eat correctly.

How This Plan Works

The most important and powerful regulatory chemicals in your body are your hormones. Hormones might very well be the single-most-important factor when it comes to weight loss. For example, the hormone insulin tells your body to store. Depending on how your body is functioning, it can tell your body to store either fat or muscle. With the lack of proper levels of intensity when training, combined with the onslaught of simple carbohydrates many people eat on a daily basis, most peoples' bodies are in prime fat-storage mode. Eating one piece of candy or one bite of cake can be enough to spike your insulin and put you into fat-storage mode. Even though you may be eating a limited amount of calories, that one little piece of candy or cake has the power to change how your body handles food in a negative way.

The key is to eat foods that better regulate and improve your insulin sensitivity. If you are going to eat carbohydrates, the idea is to eat them after a workout or training session. Eating the right carbs after the proper intensity training will get you to take advantage of your body being more insulin sensitive. When your body chemistry is optimal and you are more insulin sensitive, the carbs will be used to fill glycogen (energy) stores in your muscle and *not* your fat cells. If you follow this plan properly, even excess carbohydrates will be used to build muscle and *not* fat.

Fat loss is this simple. You want to burn the stored fat in your body, right? Well, your body's preferred source of energy is carbohydrates. If you eat carbs, your body will burn that for energy and never get to the stored fat in your body. In addition, you are spiking your levels of the hormone insulin, which tells your body to store any excess energy. Through proper intensity exercise and having a plan of when to eat carbohydrates, you will teach your body to burn stored fat as energy on a regular basis.

Through this plan you will improve hormone regulation, starting with insulin. Hormones work together in a cycle. If your lifestyle has your hormones out of whack, then insulin can also affect testosterone (which regulates the body's ability to build lean muscle) and cortisol (the stress hormone leading to more stored belly fat), thus continuing a vicious cycle that can simply not be fixed by eating smaller portions and doing some light cardio a couple times a week.

If you are trying to lose weight and are not successful even though you are eating less than 1500 to 2000 calories a day, you simply need to change your body's chemistry. Even though every individual is different, the typical individual should be able to lose fat eating this range of calories. Once you change your body's chemistry and it is functioning optimally, you will be more apt to lose fat and not muscle. This is the key to body re-composition.

The New Plan

The way to successfully cause a positive change in the body's chemistry, thus creating long-term sustained changes to physique and health, is through the proper balance of the type of food you eat and the activities that you do. The *Do This, Eat That* plan carefully creates a relationship between types of food (based on their macro-nutrient breakdown) and exercises that can be performed on a daily basis. This will change the way your body functions and turn it into a fat-burning machine.

The good news is that in this book, we have done all the work for you! Simply look up the food you are going to eat, and you will find a list of possible exercises linked to this food. If you do the suggested exercise prior to eating your chosen food, your body will have the capability to use the food more efficiently. Choose the exercise(s) that best fits your situation based on the type of food you are going to eat. If you do not like the exercise or cannot fit it into your schedule, then simply pick another food. Many foods from this list require no exercise at all!

Exercising and eating in this way helps optimize your body's chemistry right from day one of this program because your body best utilizes the effects of insulin directly after exercise. You are essentially turning every meal into a post workout meal. Because you eat multiple times in a day, this will give you a high frequency of training that is great for cutting fat and adding lean muscle.

This book also will teach you what foods are the best for achieving your goal of weight loss. You can choose a whole day's worth of meals that require no exercise at all because they are the optimal food choices for fat loss. We provide a variety of different exercises, many with modifications that fit your current fitness level. These exercises also allow for progress and advancement. Just follow the book, and your body has no choice but to achieve its body composition goals and begin functioning better immediately.

This plan consists of looking up any food you are going to eat, and based on the breakdown of the food, seeing if it requires any exercise prior to consumption. If the food requires no exercise then it is a perfect food for fat loss. If the food requires an exercise choice, then you must perform the exercise *before* you eat the food in order to keep the body in prime fat burning mode. Let's begin the process by looking at what tools you will need to reference in order to follow the plan.

Extra Credit Information....

Doing Things Right

There is a common nutritional misconception that exists regarding the right way to eat that has people struggling to hit their goals. Many people are willing to put in the effort in order to achieve their goals, but if they are misled, their efforts might be misdirected and they may never realize their goals.

Quote: "My friend is trying that fad diet where you don't eat any bread or pasta, just meat and stuff. Isn't that bad for you?" You will hear variations of this quote all over the place. You constantly hear talk in the gym that the idea of limiting carbs such as bread, pasta, and sugar is somehow a "fad diet." This couldn't be further from the truth.

First, the idea of being on a "diet" is completely blown out of proportion. A "fad diet" implies that there is a plan that you are going to follow for a short period of time to obtain fast results. This is an ineffective way to go about things long term because eventually you will fall back into the same habits you had before, thus going back to how you looked and felt before.

If you are on a "diet" people automatically assume that you are trying to lose weight. In reality being on a "diet" actually means you have a plan or a rhyme or reason to what you are eating and when you are eating it. Having a plan is extremely important to achieving a variety of goals. In this respect everyone should be on a "diet." Whether you are trying to cut fat, put on muscle, or increase your performance at a sport, you should have a plan that has you eating the correct foods at the right times.

Many individuals do have a primary objective of losing fat and getting leaner. If cutting fat and getting leaner is your primary objective, man-made processed, starchy carbs like bread, pasta, and sugar are death to fat loss. It seems as if through the years, foods like pasta and bread have been construed as being natural and healthy, whereas in reality your body does not have any dietary need for them. Your body does have a need for a diet high in quality protein, vegetables, and healthy fat. You could live for the rest of your life just eating proteins, healthy fats, and carbohydrates found solely in vegetables. In turn, if you were to just eat carbs, you would not last very long before your body began to break down.

Also in relation to this, over the years unhealthy "trans fats" have been incorrectly grouped with saturated fats and animal fats. While trans fats should be avoided, animal fats from healthy animals such as grass-fed beef, wild salmon, and coconut oil are some of the healthiest things you can eat. If you eat these fats along with proteins, you will actually promote fat loss in the body because your body becomes more efficient at burning fat for energy. Healthy fats help prevent chronic systemic inflammation that can be a primary cause of many diseases. Meanwhile the protein will keep your body's metabolic rate high because it is very thermo-genic and rebuilds and supports muscle mass.

However, when you introduce simple carbs into the equation, your body will use those for energy and store the excess as fat. This means that simple carbs are the enemy, not protein or fat. Excess carbohydrates that get broken down into sugar in the body are also the building block for triglycerides. Elevated triglycerides in the system are responsible for elevated low density lipo-proteins (bad cholesterol,) and decreased high density lipo-proteins (good cholesterol.) This is especially important because many people incorrectly correlate their poor cholesterol numbers with fats and cholesterol found in meat and eggs. In reality the dietary fat and cholesterol found in these foods work to increase HDL (Good) cholesterol, especially when choosing farm fresh cage-free eggs, or organic grass-fed beef. When people stop eating these foods (that are actually helping their cholesterol,) and replace them with foods "low" in fat and cholesterol, and high in carbohydrates, it usually results in their health issues becoming worse.

Eating a high percentage of healthy fats and proteins will also increase your body's insulin sensitivity and put you into fat-burning mode. Eating healthy fats and proteins that are found in such sources as wild caught fish, nuts, and complex carbohydrates found in vegetables like broccoli and spinach, will help fight disease, keep you regulated, better your immune system, fight inflammation, help build muscle, balance your hormones, and increase your sex drive!

CHAPTER 1: DO THIS, EAT THAT

Do This: Exercises

You will see lists of exercises broken down into categories and put together in a table. Complete descriptions and photos along with modifications and progressions for these exercises can be found further on in the book. Each exercise category is as follows and is associated with a letter:

A = light cardiovascular activity
B = light to moderate cardiovascular activity
C = moderate to high cardiovascular activity
D = light resistance activity
E = light to moderate resistance activity
F = moderate to high resistance activity

Under each column are separate exercises or groups of exercises to choose from, all of which can be modified and progressed depending on ability level. It is important to challenge yourself in order to make these effective. What exactly does this mean? When it comes to exercise, it is very important to remember that you are trying to change your body. Whether your goal is to lose weight, get stronger, or simply get healthier, the idea is to force your body into an adaptation. This means you must place new demands on it so that it will want to change. You must attempt weights and exercises that you can "barely" do, rather than exercises and weights you can do for a while or for many reps.

If you are just exercising to sweat and burn calories, you are missing out on one of the most important aspects of training. Do not place limits on yourself, and remember that if you can "barely" do something, that means you *can* do it. Force yourself to do more and more things you can "barely" do, and your body will be forced to adapt to the new circumstances, which ultimately means new levels achieved. Keep this in mind when doing your chosen exercises.

Modifications and progressions for the exercises we've listed will be explicitly shown and explained in the following pages. However, you can always follow this general rule of thumb: if after you do ten repetitions of an exercise it feels like you could do ten more, you need to add more resistance. Using the ten-repetition example, when you get to your seventh or eighth repetition, you should feel as though squeezing out those last two or three reps takes everything you've got.

Conversely, if you are unable to do ten repetitions in a row of your body weight, simply take breaks in between until you reach ten. As you progress you will notice that you will be taking fewer and fewer breaks in between until doing ten in a row is achievable.

The same goes for cardio work: if after a five-minute walk you feel the same as you did before you started, you need to pick it up a bit and perhaps run for those five minutes. If you are out of breath from walking after two minutes, slow down or stop and continue after a short break until you have done a total of five minutes of walking.

For the higher-resistance exercise choices, you can break the reps down however you would like. For instance, if you have to do thirty push-ups, you can do six sets of whatever level push-up you can do five repetitions of, with a break in between. Do not get discouraged over the exercises; we have chosen the most modifiable exercises, so no matter your level, there will always be a modification for you.

Here is the list of exercises to choose from.

A	B	C
25 jumping jacks	50 jumping jacks	75 jumping jacks
1 minute of jumping rope	2 minutes of jumping rope	3 minutes of jumping rope
10 leapfrog squats	20 leapfrog squats	30 leapfrog squats
25 mountain climbers	50 mountain climbers	75 mountain climbers
10 of each: cradle walks, Spiderman lunges, bird/dog, scapular wall slide, reach and rolls	20 plank rotations	30 jumping lunges
10 of each: squats, high knees, warrior lunges, glute/ham bridges, fire hydrant	20 plank shoulder taps	15 leapfrog squats/ kick back to plank/ push-up/repeat
5 minute walk or jog	10-minute walk or jog	15-minute walk or jog
5-minutes yoga sequence	10-minute yoga sequence	15-minute yoga sequence

D	E	F
20 body-weight squats	40 body-weight squats	60 body-weight squats
15 dumbbell rows	20 dumbbell rows	30 dumbbell rows
10 overhead presses	20 overhead presses	30 overhead presses
10 pull-ups	20 pull-ups	30 pull-ups
15 pushups	30 pushups	50 pushups
10 single leg deadlifts	20 single leg deadlifts	30 single leg deadlifts
20 sit-ups	40 sit-ups	60 sit-ups
10 walking lunges	20 walking lunges	30 walking lunges

These exercises will be described more in-depth in the chapter, *Exercises in Detail*

Eat That: Foods

In the following table, you will see six columns. You will also notice a letter (or letters) associated with each column that correlates directly to the "Do This" table. The columns list foods that are categorized by macro-nutrient ratios. Macro-nutrients are the proteins, fats and carbohydrates found in food. This is how we have broken it down. You will not need to know the macro-nutrient breakdown to follow the plan because we have indexed all the food for you. However, this does offer a reference as to the rationale behind the plan. Simply locate the food you are about to eat and see what category it falls under. Then look to see what exercises you need to do prior to eating your chosen food.

Optimal = protein/fiber: Foods that require no exercise to lose fat.
Great = protein/fiber/fat: Foods that are conducive to fat loss, but still require some light cardio prior to consumption.
Good = protein/fiber/fat/low-glycemic carbs: These are foods that are healthy and do not have a large impact on insulin. However, these foods do contain a lot of energy that has to be accounted for through some resistance exercise and light cardio prior to consumption.

Poor = protein/fiber/higher fats or higher-glycemic carbs: Foods that are not conducive to fat loss, and require more-intense resistance and cardio exercise prior to consumption.

Risky = protein/fiber/higher fats or starches (highest-glycemic carbs): Foods that require a higher volume of resistance exercise and cardio to put the body into a state of insulin sensitivity in order to properly handle this amount of carbohydrates.

Makes You Fat (MYF) = high sugar/high fat/high starch: Foods that should only be consumed on special occasions. On these special occasions, they require the highest levels of exercise prior to consumption in order to prime your body best to handle them. Due to the combination of fat and carbs in the foods in this category, these foods are death to fat loss without proper exercise first. The primary goal when eating or drinking foods from this category is to not take any steps backward from your fat-loss goals. Proper exercise will help to maintain the progress you have made and allow you to keep moving forward without any huge setbacks.

Optimal	Great (A)	Good (A & D)
green vegetables	nuts	yogurt, greek (plain)
fish	natural peanut butter	beans
poultry	avocados	peanut butter
meat	cheese	hummus
eggs	soups or stews with no starches	milk fat-free
beef jerky (non-sweetened)	lentils	butter
protein powder	protein shakes (10 grams of carbs or less)	sour cream
water, tea, coffee	protein bars (10 grams of carbs or less)	dressings: blue cheese, ranch
non-sweetened drinks	dark chocolate (80 percent or higher)	
artificial sweeteners	olives	
mustard	mayonnaise	
vinegar	oils	
any spices		

Poor (B & E)	Risky (C & E)	Make You Fat (C & F)
fruits/berries	pasta, plain	rice, flavored
corn	sauces	yogurts, flavored
squash	rice	oatmeal, flavored
carrots	bread (breading)	pizza
tofu/meat substitute	cereal	desserts
protein bars (more than 10 grams of carbs)	potatoes	jellies
oatmeal	soups or stews with starches	fruit juices
milk 1 percent or higher	pretzels	all sugary beverages
tomatoes	crackers	alcohol
tomato sauce	tortilla chips	
ketchup		
balsamic vinegar		
dark chocolate (60–79 percent)		

We have kept these lists relatively short and general for ease of use. Provided here is an elaboration on some of the more general foods; you can also find a more comprehensive list further on in the book. If you cannot find your food on here, you can also compare it to a food of similar macro-nutrient breakdown to get your letter.

- **Green vegetables** includes spinach, kale, collard greens, swiss chard, turnip greens, mustard greens, broccoli, red/green-leaf and romaine lettuce, cabbage, iceberg lettuce, peppers, and celery.
- **Fish** includes any fish such as cod, haddock, salmon, tuna, shrimp, and scallops.
- **Meats** includes chicken, turkey, beef, lamb, pork, bacon, sausage, and lunchmeat.
- **Nuts/seeds** includes peanuts, almonds, walnuts, cashews, and sunflower seeds.
- **Bread** includes any bread at all, even whole wheat or whole grain.
- **Rice** includes all rice, white, brown, and wild. Although some might consider whole-wheat bread and brown rice "healthier" options, they have about the same macro-nutrient breakdown as the "white" versions and will be of the same detriment to your weight-loss success.
- **Oils** includes any oils such as olive oil, canola oil, corn oil, vegetable oil, and peanut oil.
- **Desserts** includes pretty much *any* sugar at all such as cake, pie, ice cream, puddings, cookies, milk chocolate, and sugar candy.

- **Alcohol** includes any alcohol at all. Although there are different amounts of carbohydrates in different alcohols, alcohol itself has a negative effect on blood sugar and insulin.

Extra Credit Information.....

The Top Eight Foods You Should Be Eating Every Week

No matter what your goals are, here are the top eight foods you should be eating every week to make sure you are maximizing your progress.

Free-range chicken or grass-fed beef: Most of your meals should be centered on these meats which contain all the protein you need.

Wild-caught deep-sea fish like cod and salmon: The benefits of eating fish are widely known, but buying fish that is wild caught will ensure maximum levels of omega-3, and getting deep-sea fish will minimize mercury levels.

Broccoli: This vegetable is nutrient rich and full of fiber. Eat steamed or raw for maximum levels of nutrition, but don't be afraid to season with your favorite spices and some extra-virgin olive oil.

Farm-fresh eggs: Cook them however you want, eat the whole egg, and good things will happen.

Almonds: These nuts are packed with minerals, protein, and fiber.

Ninety to one hundred percent dark cocoa: This is simply one of the highest-antioxidant foods you can eat.

Dark red kidney beans: These beans are filled with nutrients, protein, and fiber. These are a high energy food, and according to the *Do This, Eat That* plan, require some exercise before consumption.

Berries: Try to eat them post-workout because of the high levels of sugar, but they contain tons of vitamins and minerals that produce healthy chemical responses in the body; for example, they provide a buffer that helps fight acidity.

CHAPTER 2: MAKE IT HAPPEN

You have now been given the tools to put the plan into action, so it's time to begin. You will need to consult the two tables in the previous chapter before you eat. Decide on what you are going to eat at the time, find that food on the food chart, and see what letter(s) match up to it. Then, under that letter column, find one exercise per each different food that you eat that fits into what you are able to do at that time, and perform it before you eat your chosen food.

It is extremely important to remember that *quantity* of one specific food does not matter. For example, if you are planning to eat pasta, you must perform one exercise from category C and one exercise from category E. Once you perform those exercises, you can eat as much of that specific pasta as you would like. However, if you were going to eat pasta and also another food from the "Risky" category such as some bread, you would have to do another set of exercises from categories C and E. If you were to pick another food to eat from another category, you would have to choose another exercise or exercises to do.

Here is how it works:

Meal Example

Food	Food Category	Exercise Category
eggs	Optimal	none
feta cheese	Great	A
toast	Risky	C & E

Using the tables from page 4 and 7, one exercise routine option for this meal would be as follows: you could do thirty push-ups (C), twenty-five jumping jacks (A), and three minutes of jumping rope (C). Again, ideally this should be done right before you eat. This will help prep your body to handle the food it's about to take in as efficiently as possible.   Also, when given the opportunity try to do resistance exercises before cardiovascular exercises. This is not mandatory; however it will promote optimal body composition.

Take note as to how realistically you could do this at home in the morning before you eat breakfast; this routine would take you less than ten minutes to accomplish. If you're not in the mood to jump rope or do push-ups, then just don't eat the toast! You could even fill up on a few more eggs, and you would not have to do more exercises.

You will notice that we have not focused on portion size. This plan is more concerned with the macronutrient breakdown and how the body processes those nutrients.

If you follow this plan and begin to make the association between your nutrient intake and intensity of exercise, you will begin to make the right food choices overall for fat loss. If you know, for example, that you will be stuck in the office all day with little or no time to perform any of these exercises, you will be more apt to choose food items from the Optimal or Great categories. It is also important to note that this plan should be added to your normal daily activities or training. To optimize fat loss, avoid making substitutions for the exercises on your own, and try to stick to the plan. An active lifestyle will help you further achieve your fat loss goals, but only if you are complying with the basic fundamentals of the *Do This, Eat That* plan.

An example of what this might look like is as follows:

Daily Meal Plan Example

Meal 1

Food	Food Category	Exercise Category
oatmeal	Poor	B & E
banana	Risky	C & E
black coffee	Optimal	none

20 walking lunges during your 10-minute walk, 75 jumping jacks, and 30 push-ups

Meal 2

Food	Food Category	Exercise Category
protein powder with water	Optimal	none
broccoli	Optimal	none
hummus	Good	A & D

5-minutes yoga and 20 sit-ups

Meal 3

Food	Food Category	Exercise Category
spinach salad with....	Optimal	none
grilled chicken	Optimal	none
bacon	Optimal	none
apple-cider vinegar	Optimal	none
diet soda	Optimal	none

No exercise needed prior to meal

Meal 4

Food	Food Category	Exercise Category
natural peanut butter	Great	A
celery	Optimal	none

1 minute of jumping rope

Meal 5

Food	Food Category	Exercise Category
salmon	Optimal	none
spinach sautéed with...	Optimal	none
cooking spay	Optimal	none
garlic salt	Optimal	none
brown rice	Risky	C & E

15 jumping lunges and 40 sit-ups

You will notice that this meal plan has you eating five times throughout the day and exercising a total of approximately thirty minutes. You can vary this so that you are eating only three or four times a day if you'd prefer. Again, this plan is focused on the correlation between exercise and food intake and not necessarily portion or frequency of eating. As long as you can do the exercises associated with the food you are about to eat, you are all set.

Extra Credit Information.....

Foods People Love That Aren't as Bad for You as You Might Think

1. **Cheese:** Cheese has gotten a bad rap over the years. Though it is relatively high in calories, it is high in protein with close to zero carbs. As part of a low-carb, fat-loss plan, cheese can be a very good food choice. If you are really concerned with the calories, try a reduced or non-fat option.

2. **Bacon:** This is another food that people always associate with being not healthy for some reason. It has no carbs and is high in protein. It is also relatively easy to cook off a large portion of the fat and grease if you are trying to limit calories. This is a much better food choice than all those cereals, yogurts, and "whole-wheat" breads individuals traditionally eat for breakfast.

3. **Eggs:** There is a misconception that eggs will send your cholesterol levels through the roof. Actually, eggs (especially farm-fresh, cage-free eggs) are loaded with healthy fat and cholesterol that can have a positive effect on your health.

4. **Nuts:** People usually dwell on the fact that nuts are high in fat. Well, the first thing to know is that eating fat doesn't make you fat; eating sugar does. Nuts are high in healthy omega

fats. Omega fatty acids are healthy for just about every body system, along with helping to fight many diseases. Eating a diet high in healthy fats can ensure proper hormone levels, fight inflammation, and help you to lose weight.

Sample Seven-Day Meal Plan

Now that you understand how to use the two tables, we've provided you with a sample food plan for the week, comprised mostly of Optimal and Great foods for fat loss. After each meal the food and exercise category is marked. You will notice that this is a rather simple plan. This was done purposely to show that even when you are minimally active, weight loss can be achieved healthily and without losing muscle.

The more active you become the greater variety of foods you have to choose from, and so many more options open up for you. Remember, you can eat almost anything you want on occasion; you just need to prep your body properly before doing so if you are looking to lose fat.

Monday

8 a.m. **(A)** 2 scoops protein with cinnamon, flaxseed oil, and water

12 p.m. **(A)x2** Salad with grilled or pan-cooked chicken, cheese, and black olives, seasoned with olive oil and apple-cider vinegar

4 p.m. **(A)** 1 serving mixed nuts

8 p.m. **(A)** Wild-caught Alaskan cod seasoned with red pepper, sea salt, turmeric spice, and olive oil, baked in the oven; steamed broccoli seasoned with olive oil and sea salt

Tuesday

8 a.m. **(A)** 2 scoops protein with cinnamon, flaxseed oil, and water

12 p.m. **(A)** Tuna-and-cheese lettuce wrap

4 p.m. **(A)** 1 serving of mixed nuts

8 p.m. **(A)** Grass-fed steak seasoned with sea salt and turmeric spice, steamed spinach seasoned with olive oil and sea salt

Wednesday

8 a.m. **(A)** 2 scoops protein with cinnamon, flaxseed oil, and water

12 p.m. **(A)** Beef and vegetable soup

4 p.m. **(A)** 1 serving mixed nuts

8 p.m. **(A)x2** Chicken stir-fry with a cut up onion, peppers, and mushrooms (put it all in pan with water and cook until water evaporates out); 90 percent dark chocolate and natural peanut butter (Smart Balance, chunky or creamy)

Thursday

8 a.m. **(A)** 2 scoops protein with cinnamon, flaxseed oil, and water

12 p.m. **(A)x2** Salad with salmon or tuna, fat-free cheese, and black olives, seasoned with olive oil and apple-cider vinegar

4 p.m. **(A)** 1 serving mixed nuts

8 p.m. **(A)** Farm-fresh eggs scrambled with spinach and avocado

Friday

8 a.m. **(A)** 2 scoops protein with cinnamon, flaxseed oil, and water

12 p.m. **(A)** Salad with grilled or pan-cooked chicken, fat-free cheese, and black olives, seasoned with olive oil

4 p.m. **(A)** 1 serving mixed nuts

8 p.m. **(A)(A/D)** Wild-caught Alaskan cod seasoned with red pepper, sea salt, turmeric, and olive oil and baked in the oven; dark-red kidney beans heated and seasoned with sea salt and olive oil

Saturday

8 a.m. **(A)** 2 scoops protein with cinnamon, flaxseed oil, and water

12 p.m. **(A)x2** Eggs any way with green beans seasoned with sea salt and olive oil, avocado, and bacon

8 p.m. **(A)x2** Salad with salmon or tuna, fat-free cheese, and black olives, seasoned with olive oil

Sunday

8 a.m. **(A)** 2 scoops protein with cinnamon, flaxseed oil, and water

12 p.m. **(A)x2** Eggs any way with green beans seasoned with sea salt and olive oil, avocado, and bacon

8 p.m. **(None)** Chicken breast and broccoli/cauliflower mix seasoned with whatever spices you like

*Every day drink as much non-sweetened green tea as possible! Green tea is a great way to boost metabolism and is high in antioxidants.

If you were to break down the exercises per day in this meal plan, you are looking at needing to be active approximately ten to fifteen minutes a day. Given the fact that most of us are awake roughly sixteen hours a day, those fifteen minutes add up to only 1.5 percent of your day. In a nutshell, if you are looking to lose weight, this plan makes that very possible, even if you are not a workout fanatic.

The Optimal category foods make a great list to shop from! Fill your house with the "Optimal" foods in the list below, and you will be well on your way to positively changing your body composition.

The following pages provide you with a log worksheet and easy to carry around version of the *Do This, Eat That* charts to help you maximize your adherence and accountability.

What I need to do before...   *...I eat this.*

Exercise	Category

>>>
>>>
>>>
>>>
>>>
>>>
>>>
>>>
>>>
>>>
>>>
>>>
>>>
>>>
>>>
>>>
>>>
>>>
>>>
>>>
>>>
>>>
>>>

Food	Category

Exercises

A	B	C
25 jumping jacks	50 jumping jacks	75 jumping jacks
1 minute of jumping rope	2 minutes of jumping rope	3 minutes of jumping rope
10 leapfrog squats	20 leapfrog squats	30 leapfrog squats
25 mountain climbers	50 mountain climbers	75 mountain climbers
10 of each: cradle walks, Spiderman lunges, bird/dogs, scapular wall slides, reach and rolls	20 plank rotations	30 jumping lunges
10 of each: squats, high knees, warrior lunges, glute/ham bridges, fire hydrants	20 plank shoulder taps	15 leapfrog squats/kick back to plank/push-up/repeat
5 minute walk or jog	10-minute walk or jog	15-minute walk or jog
5-minute yoga sequence	10-minute yoga sequence	15-minute yoga sequence

D	E	F
20 body-weight squats	40 body-weight squats	60 body-weight squats
15 dumbbell rows	20 dumbbell rows	30 dumbbell rows
10 overhead presses	20 overhead presses	30 overhead presses
10 pull-ups	20 pull-ups	30 pull-ups
15 pushups	30 pushups	50 pushups
10 single leg deadlifts	20 single leg deadlifts	30 single leg deadlifts
20 sit-ups	40 sit-ups	60 sit-ups
10 walking lunges	20 walking lunges	30 walking lunges

Foods

Optimal	Great (A)	Good (A & D)
green vegetables	nuts	yogurt, greek (plain)
fish	natural peanut butter	beans
poultry	avocados	peanut butter
meat	cheese	hummus
eggs	soups or stews with no starches	milk fat-free
beef jerky	lentils	butter
protein powder	protein shakes (10 grams of carbs or less)	sour cream
water, tea, coffee	protein bars (10 grams of carbs or less)	dressings: blue cheese, ranch
unsweetened drinks	dark chocolate (80 percent or higher)	
artificial sweeteners	olives	
mustard	mayonnaise	
vinegar	oils	
any spices		

Poor (B & E)	Risky (C & E)	Make You Fat (C & F)
fruits	pasta, plain	rice, flavored
corn	lentils	yogurts, flavored
squash	rice	oatmeal, flavored
carrots	bread	pizza
tofu/meat substitute	cereal	desserts
protein bars (more than 10 grams of carbs)	potatoes	jellies
oatmeal	soups or stews with starches	fruit juices
milk 1 percent or higher	pretzels	all sugary beverages
tomatoes	crackers	alcohol
tomato sauce	tortilla chips	
Ketchup		
balsamic vinegar		
dark chocolate (60–79 percent)		

CHAPTER 3: EXERCISES IN DETAIL

The following pages provide you with photos and step-by-step descriptions as to how to execute many of the exercises or series of exercises listed in chapter one, along with modifications and progressions. You will be given a brief explanation as to how to adjust some of these exercises to fit your ability level. You will also find that each exercise is referenced to an article or articles from the appendix that will provide you with more detailed information regarding that specific exercise.

Bird/Dogs
(Reference "Flexibility Versus Stability" pg. 75)

Start in a tabletop position with hands and knees on the floor. Hands are directly underneath your shoulders and knees directly underneath your hips. Keep your head and neck in alignment with your spine by looking down at the floor with your chin tucked. Activate your abdominals, squeeze your glutes, and then lift your right leg and extend it straight back in line with your torso; at the same time extend your left arm forward, also keeping it in line with your torso. Hold for two seconds then draw both back down to the floor, all while keeping your glutes and midsection engaged. Then extend the opposite pair.

Modification: Do not use the arms; only do the leg extensions.
Progression: Do this from a plank position rather than tabletop.

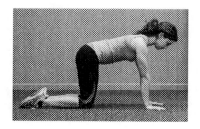 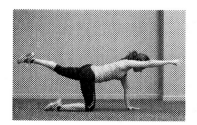

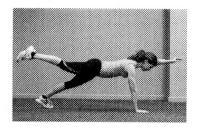

Cradle Walks

(Reference "Correct Posture When Performing Exercises" pg. 74 and "Flexibility Versus Stability" pg. 75)

Standing straight, shift weight onto your left leg, grab the instep of your right foot, and pull upward with both hands. Your hip will rotate externally as your knee bends; gently continue to pull your leg upward while keeping your shoulders down and away from your ears without rounding your back. Release your right leg, step forward, and repeat on your left.

Modification: Go slowly and use a balance assist such as a wall or chair.
Progression: Jump between each transition.

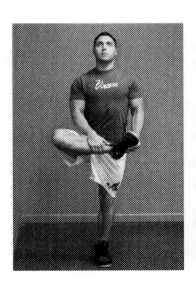
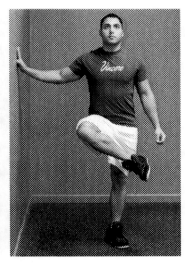

Dumbbell Rows

(Reference "Correct Posture When Performing Exercises" pg. 74 and "Proper Shoulder Function" pg. 76)

Kneel over the side of a bench by placing your knee and hand of one supporting arm on the bench. Position the foot of your opposite leg slightly back and to the side. Grasp dumbbell from floor.

Pull dumbbell up to your side until your upper arm is just beyond horizontal. Then bring dumbbell down so that your arm is extended and your shoulder is stretched downward. Repeat and continue with your opposite arm.

Modification: Pull dumbbell up as high as you can.
Progression: Use heavier weights.

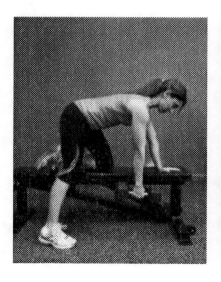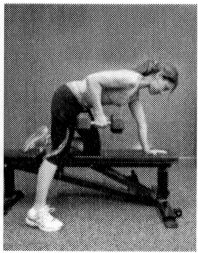

Fire Hydrants
(Reference "Flexibility Versus Stability" pg. 75)

Begin in a tabletop position with hands and feet on the floor. Wrists should be directly below your shoulders and knees below your hips, creating a ninety-degree angle in the legs. Keeping this ninety-degree angle, raise one leg out to the side, trying to get your knee to the same level as your hips; squeeze and hold for a count of one, then slowly bring the leg down to the starting position. Repeat on the opposite side.

Modification: Go only as far as tolerated without shifting your body.
Progression: Work through a full range of motion.

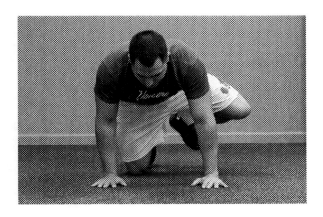

Glute/Ham Bridges
(Reference "Flexibility Versus Stability" pg. 75)

Lie on your back with your legs bent, knees up and feet flat on the floor. Squeeze your glutes, and lift your hips up to the sky. Hold and squeeze at the top of this movement, then slowly return to the starting position. Do not raise your hips too high; this will create a curvature or hyperextension of your lumbar spine.

> Modification: Only go as high as you can while maintaining form and even force on legs.
> Progression: Raise one leg and perform the same motion, making sure both hips are always even during every stage of the movement.

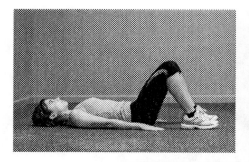
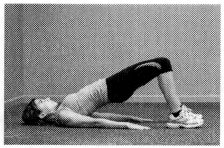
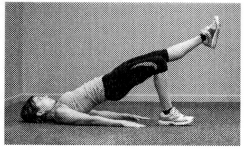

High Knees
(Reference "Correct Posture When Performing Exercises" pg.74 and "Flexibility Versus Stability" pg. 75)

Standing straight, bend your right leg and lift your knee to your chest. With both hands clasp your right leg directly under your knee, draw your leg toward your chest, and hold for one count. Release leg, step forward, and repeat on left side. Keep an upright posture with chin tucked while going through this movement.

Modification: Go slowly and use a balance assist such as a wall or chair.
Progression: Jump between each transition.

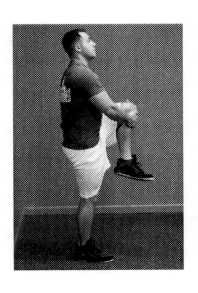 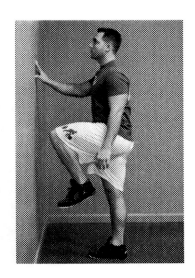

Jumping Jacks

(Reference "Correct Posture When Performing Exercises" pg. 74)

Stand with your arms at your sides. Be sure your feet are straight and close together. Hold your head straight.

Bend your knees. Jump up while spreading your arms and legs at the same time. Lift your arms to your ears, and open your feet to a little wider than shoulder width in a fluid movement. Clap or touch your hands above your head. As you return from jumping up, bring your arms back down to your sides, and at the same time bring your feet back together.

Modification: Perform without jumping, going as slowly as you need.
Progression: Jump as high as possible and go faster.

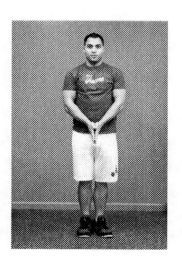
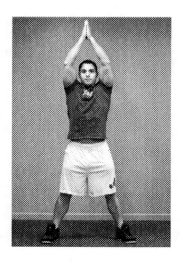

Jumping Rope
(Reference "Correct Posture When Performing Exercises" pg. 74)

Find a jump rope that fits your height: Hold each end in each one of your hands, stepping on the rope making sure each side is even. The handles should fit right under your armpits.

Holding on to the handles, stand in front of the rope. Begin by rotating your wrists and bringing the rope overhead; when it comes around, jump over it.

Modification: Go slowly, resting as much as you need.
Progression: Jump as high as possible and go faster, or try double jumps.

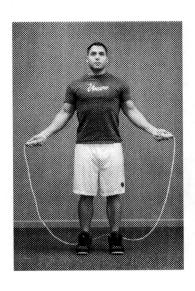 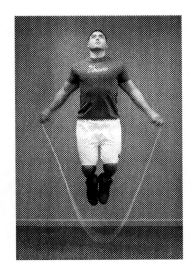

Leapfrog Squats

(Reference "Squat Mechanics for the Beginner" pg. 83)

Place your feet wider than hip width apart, bend your knees, and lower your hips toward the ground, placing all weight onto the heels of your feet.

Continue lowering until your knees are as close to a ninety-degree angle as possible. Stay in this position as you touch the ground between your legs and jump up.

> Modification: Either do not jump or make a small jump.
> Progression: Jump as high as possible.

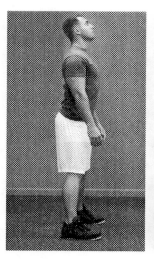
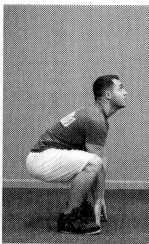
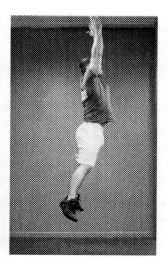

Mountain Climbers
(Reference "Correct Posture When Performing Exercises"
pg. 74)

Begin in a plank/push-up position. Keep the weight on the
balls of your feet while bringing your right leg forward to
your chest and quickly back to its original position. While
the right leg thrusts back, the left comes forward. Repeat
this motion.

Modification: Place hands on a wall or bench.
Progression: Go from the ground and speed up the
movement.

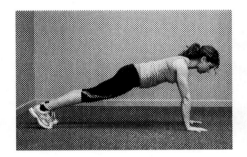 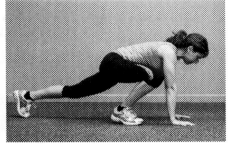

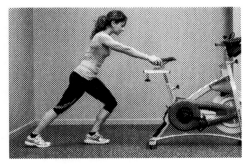

Overhead Presses

(Reference "Correct Posture When Performing Exercises"
pg. 74 and "Proper Shoulder Function" pg. 76)

Begin in a standing position. Start with two dumbbells
at a weight you can safely lift over your head. Stand
with your feet hip width apart and pick up the weights,
holding the dumbbells so your palms are facedown. Lift
up your weights until they are at your shoulders, palms
facing forward, with elbows bent at a ninety-degree
angle. Raise your arms until your elbows are extended,
moving the weights until they almost touch above your
head. Slowly return to starting position (with elbows at a
ninety-degree angle).

> Modification: Do this seated in a chair with back sup-
> port using just your arms.
> Progression: Use as much weight as you can do,
> using your entire body to help power weight up.

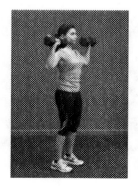
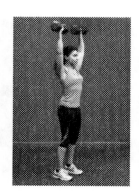
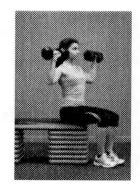

Plank Rotations
(Reference "Correct Posture When Performing Exercises"
pg. 74 and "Flexibility Versus Stability" pg. 75)

Begin in a plank position with your hands flat on the floor
directly below your shoulders. From the back of your head
to your heels you should be in a straight line. Take your
left hand and place it a few inches in from your shoulder.
Putting your weight into that left hand, raise your right
hand up to the sky and twist right, stacking your feet.
Hold for a count and return to plank. Do the same thing
but on the other side.

Modification: Place hands on bench or chair.
Progression: While in side plank, raise the leg that is
on top by squeezing your abductor and lifting your leg.

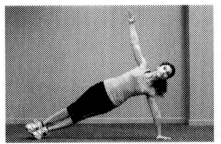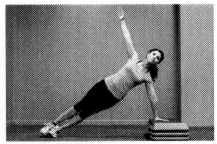
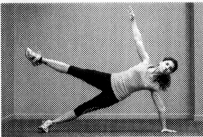

Plank Shoulder Taps

(Reference "Correct Posture When Performing Exercises" pg. 74 and "Flexibility Versus Stability" pg. 75)

Begin in a plank position with your hands flat on the floor directly below your shoulders. From the back of your head to your heels you should be in a straight line. Shift your weight slightly onto your right side, lift your left hand, and tap your right shoulder. Return your left hand to the floor, and shift your weight to the left, and lifting your right hand and tapping your left shoulder. Repeat.

Modification: Place hands on bench or chair.
Progression: While in plank keep one leg elevated and switch halfway into set.

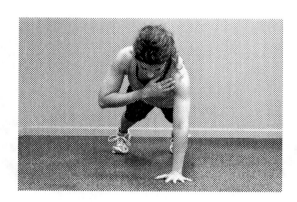

Pull-Ups
(Reference "Progressing Pull-ups" pg. 97)

Placing your hands on an overhead bar, pull yourself up so that your chin goes over the bar.

> Modification: Place the bar so that when you are standing and your arms are holding the bar, you reach the ground with your arms slightly bent. Jump up while pulling to get your chin above the bar. If the bar is high, use a bench or chair to create the above starting position.
>
> Progression: Work to a full range in which you can hit your chest to the bar; add weight by holding a dumb-bell between your legs or wearing a weighted vest.

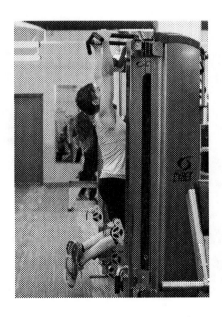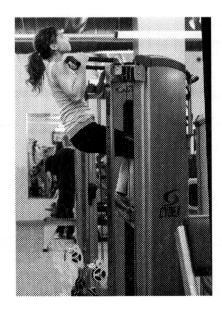

Push-Ups

(Reference "Proper Push-Ups" pg. 78)

Place your toes and hands on the floor, making sure your back and arms are straight. Keep your hands slightly more than shoulder width apart, and tighten your abdominal muscles. Lower yourself to the floor and press yourself back up.

> Modification: Place your hands on an elevated surface such as a bench or chair.
> Progression: Raise your feet up so they are elevated and you are in an incline position.

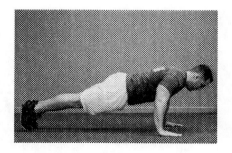 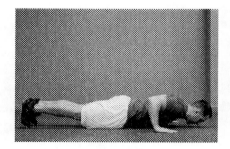

Reach and Rolls

(Reference "Flexibility Versus Stability" pg. 75 and "Proper Shoulder Function" pg. 76)

Kneel on the floor and place your forearms on the floor with your elbows in close to your knees. Slide one arm out until it is fully extended with your hand in a neutral position (thumb facing up). Once arm is fully extended, turn palm up and lift arm up without shifting torso.

Modification: Extend your arm out as far as possible while maintaining proper form.
Progression: Once full range is achieved, lift palm up toward ceiling and lift arm as far as possible without breaking form or shifting body.

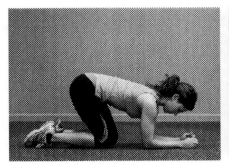 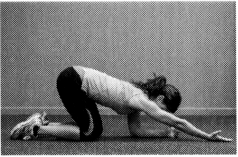

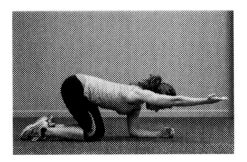

Scapular Wall Slides

(Reference "Correct Posture When Performing Exercises" pg. 74 and "Proper Shoulder Function" pg. 76)

Standing with your back against a wall, walk your feet out about twelve inches away from the wall. Lift both arms overhead and hold them back against the wall behind you. Keeping your chin tucked and head and back flat against the wall, push your elbows against the wall as you slide them down. Squeeze your shoulder blades down in the bottom position for a count of one and then repeat. Both hands and elbows should stay pressed against the wall during this movement.

Modification: Only go as far as you can keeping hands and butt touching the wall.

Progression: Work through the entire range of motion.

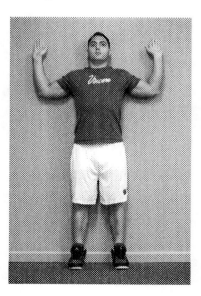 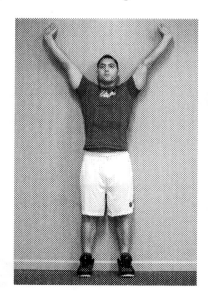

Single-Leg Dead Lifts
(Reference "Squat Mechanics for the Beginner" pg. 83)

Stand balancing on your right leg, place your left leg out behind you with your toe lightly touching the floor, or lift it completely off the floor for more of a challenge. Keeping your shoulders back, look up, holding your abs in and keeping your back flat. With a slight bend in the supporting leg, keeping your knee at the same angle throughout the movement, tip from the hips and lower the weights toward the floor. Lower as far as your flexibility allows. You can bend your knee slightly if you need to. Return to standing and repeat until desired repetitions are met, then switch legs.

Modification: Keep both feet planted firmly on the ground.
Progression: Use weights.

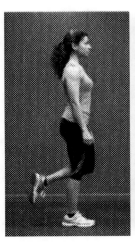 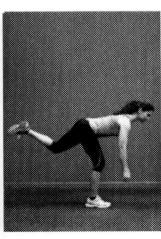 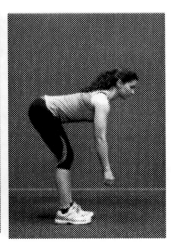

Sit-Ups

(Reference "Correct Posture When Performing Exercises" pg. 74)

Lie on your back. Bend your knees and place your feet flat on the floor. Position your heels about a foot in front of your tailbone. Place your hands behind your head loosely or cross them on your chest. Squeeze your shoulder blades together. Tighten your abs and relax your neck. Keep your head in line with your spine, but allow your head and chin to move forward a little bit as you curl up toward your bent knees. Keep the bottom of your feet, your lower back, and your tailbone flat against the floor throughout the exercise. Curl toward your thighs only until your upper back is off the mat. Slowly, and with control, lower yourself until your upper back is in contact with the floor. Repeat.

Modification: Come up only as high as possible.
Progression: Work through a full range, and add weight by holding it with arms in front of you, on your chest, or behind your head for most challenging.

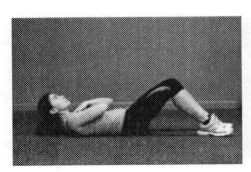
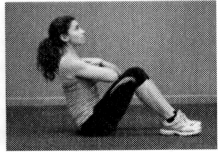

Spiderman Lunges
(Reference "Proper Lunges" pg. 91)

From a standing position, lunge forward with your right leg slightly out to the side, and sink deeply into the lunge. Keeping your chest up, place both hands flat on the floor directly below your shoulders on the inside of your right forward leg, pressing your hips down to the floor. Drive off the front foot and return to standing. Repeat on your left side and continue in a walking manner.

> Modification: Go only as low as you can while maintaining a neutral spine and keeping your knees behind your feet, using assistance for balance such as a wall or chair.
> Progression: Use a full range, and come up explosively.

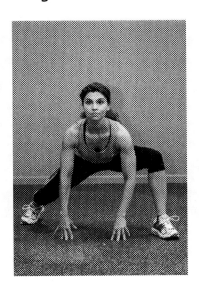 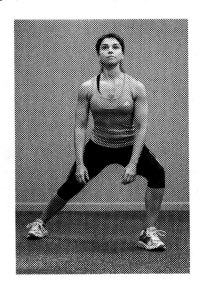

Squats

(Reference "Squat Mechanics for the Beginner" pg. 83)

Start in a standing position and sit back, keeping all your weight pushing back and into your heels. Lower yourself so that your quads are parallel to the ground and your knees are no further forward than the balls of your feet. Press through your heels and bring yourself back up to standing.

> Modification: Use the highest-level surface to squat to that you need.
> Progression: Perform a full squat with hips dropping below your knees; add weight by holding dumbbells, kettlebells, a barbell, etc.

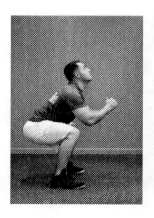 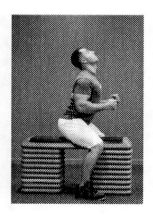 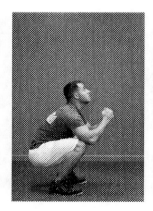

Walk or Run

(Reference "Optimal Gait" pg. 89 and "Correct Posture When Performing Exercises" pg. 74)

Modification: Walk.

Progression: Perform intervals of walking or running mixed in with sprints. Intervals are short bouts of high-intensity work coupled with lower-intensity work.

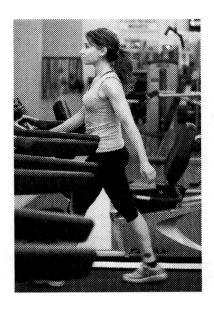
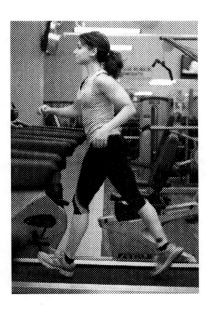

Walking Lunges

(Reference "Proper Lunges" pg. 91)

Begin in a standing position. Lunge forward with your right leg. Lower your hips down while bending both knees; your right knee should not go past the toes of that leg while keeping the weight in the heel. The knee of your left leg should come down to the ground as close as possible. Drive through your right foot and bring your left to meet your right as you stand up. Continue by lunging now with the left leg, and repeat.

> Modification: Go only as low as you can while maintaining a neutral spine and keeping your knees behind toes, using assistance for balance such as a wall or chair if needed.
> Progression: Use a full range, and come up explosively; use added weight.

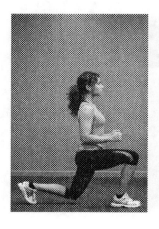 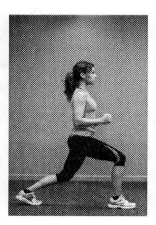 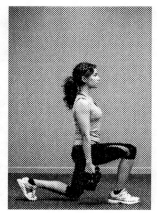

Warrior Lunges
(Reference "Proper Lunges" pg. 91)

Kneel in a lunge position, keeping your front knee over your ankle and your back knee on the ground. Stretch your arms overhead, keeping your head and chest up. Let your hips sink down, and shift your weight forward, feeling the stretch in the hip of the leg whose knee is on the ground. Hold and repeat on the opposite side.

Modification: Go only as low as you can while maintaining a neutral spine and keeping your knees behind toes, using assistance for balance such as a wall or chair.
Progression: Use a full range, and come up explosively.

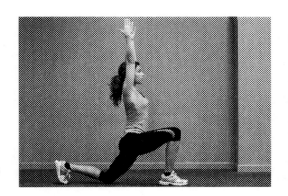
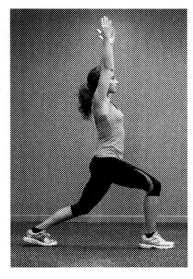

Yoga Series- Five Minute Segment

(Reference "Correct Posture When Performing Exercises" pg. 74 and "Flexibility Versus Stability" pg. 75)

The five-minute series follows this progression, as illustrated below: plank, up dog, down dog, crescent lunge, plank, up dog, down dog, crescent lunge, and plank.

Plank: Begin by placing your hands flat on the floor. Make sure your wrists are directly under your shoulders at a ninety-degree angle. Your body should be in one line from the top of your head to your heels. Do not dip or raise your hips. This is the same positioning as a push-up. Push back through your heels and forward through a neutral neck out through the top of the head. At the same time, press firmly down through your whole hand, and do not let your chest sink.

> Modification: Place your knees on the ground, keeping a straight diagonal line from your head down to your knees, the same position as a modified push-up. Progression: Lift one leg parallel to the ground.

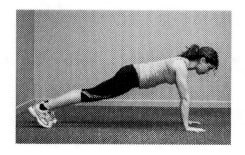
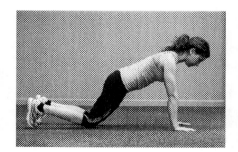

Up Dog: Lie on your stomach. Stretch your legs back and place the palms of your hands on the floor next to your shoulders, with the tops of your feet on the floor. Press through the palms of your hands while lifting your chest and simultaneously straightening your arms. Make sure to be pressing the shoulders down away from your ears and keeping your head in alignment with your neck.

Modification: Place your forearms, rather than the palms of your hands, on the ground and press up. Progression: Curl your toes under and lift your body a few inches off the ground as you press up.

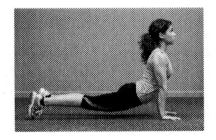
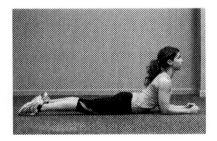

Down Dog: Begin on your hands and knees. Your wrists should be underneath your shoulders and your knees underneath your hips. Tuck your toes under your heels. Then lift your hips, coming into an upside-down V shape. Spread your fingers wide, and create a straight line between your middle fingers and elbows. Work on straightening your legs and lowering your heels toward the ground. Your heels should be slightly wider than your toes, so the outside edges of your feet are parallel with the outside edges of your mat. Relax your head between your arms, and direct your gaze through your legs or up toward your belly button.

Modification: Bend your knees.
Progression: Lift one leg up in the air while keeping your hips even and in line with one another.

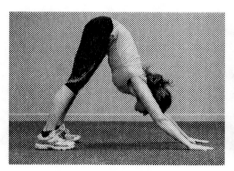 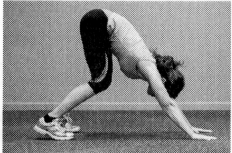

Crescent Lunge: Keep your upper body straight with your shoulders back and relaxed. Step forward with one leg, lowering your hips until your front knee is bent at about a ninety-degree angle. Make sure that your knee is above your ankle and not pushed out too far. Bring one hand down on each side of your front foot. Extend your arms forward and lift up, reaching toward the sky.

Modification: Keep your back knee down on the ground.
Progression: Sink deeper into the lunge, pressing your hips to the ground.

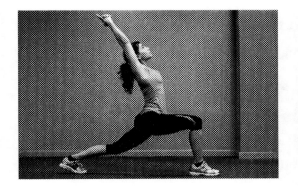
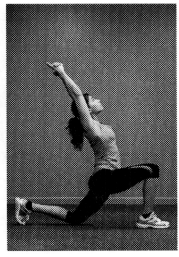

Yoga Series-Ten Minute Segment

(Reference "Correct Posture When Performing Exercises" pg. 74 and "Flexibility Versus Stability" pg. 75)

Same as five-minute series with this addition following the crescent lunge:

Knee-to-Elbow Pulls: In a plank position, draw one knee out to the side and toward your elbow. Your hips should remain level with your knee.

> Modification: Perform the same movement on your knees.
> Progression: Perform a push-up each time you draw the knee to elbow.

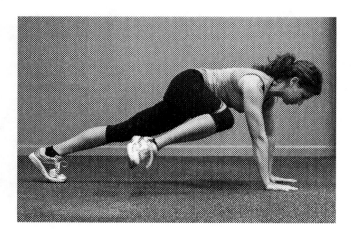

Yoga Series- Fifteen Minute Segment
(Reference "Correct Posture When Performing Exercises" pg. 74 and "Flexibility Versus Stability" pg. 75)

Same as ten-minute series with these additions following the knee-to-elbow pulls:

Knee-to-Chest Jump: In a plank position, keeping your hands on the floor, jump your feet in between your hands then back out again, and repeat.

> Modification: Walk your legs in between your hands and back out again.
> Progression: When you've completed your first jump and your legs are between your hands, jump straight up to the sky, lifting a few inches off the ground; return hands to floor and jump legs back into plank position.

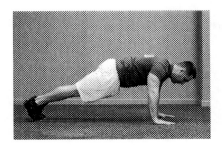 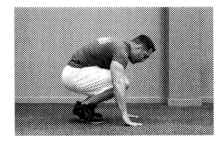

Spinal Twist: Sitting with legs extended forward, bend right leg and place your foot as close to your body as possible, knee pointing up. Bring your right arm behind you while your left comes around the right side of your right leg as you twist right, keeping your spine extended upward. Repeat on the left.

Modification: Only twist to the range you feel comfortable.
Progression: Bind the supporting arm around your body and grab under the thigh of the bent leg.

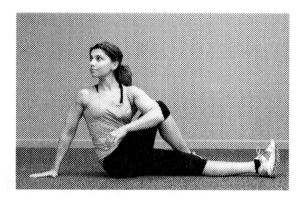

CHAPTER 4: FOODS IN DETAIL

Alphabetized List of Foods

Food Category	Vegetables	Exercise Category
Optimal	alfalfa sprouts	none
Optimal	artichoke	none
Optimal	asparagus	none
Optimal	asparagus spears	none
Optimal	bamboo shoots	none
Optimal	beans, string	None
Optimal	beets	none
Optimal	broccoli	none
Optimal	brussels sprouts	none
Optimal	cabbage	none
Poor	carrots	B & E
Poor	carrot juice	B & E
Poor	ketchup	B & E
Optimal	cauliflower	none
Optimal	celery	none
Optimal	collard greens	none
Poor	cranberry sauce, canned	B & E
Optimal	cucumber	none
Optimal	dandelion greens	none
Optimal	eggplant	none
Optimal	beans, green	none
Optimal	kale	none
Optimal	lettuce	none
Optimal	mixed greens dinner salad	none
Optimal	mushrooms	none

Optimal	mustard greens	none
Optimal	okra	none
Optimal	onion	none
Optimal	peas	none
Optimal	pepper, sweet green and red	none
Poor	pumpkin, canned	B & E
Poor	salsa	B & E
Optimal	sauerkraut	none
Great	soup, minestrone	A
Optimal	spinach	none
Poor	squash, summer	B & E
Optimal	swiss chard	none
Poor	tomato	B & E
Poor	tomato juice	B & E
Poor	tomato sauce	B & E
Optimal	turnips	none
Poor	V-8 juice	B & E
Optimal	water chestnuts	none
Optimal	watercress	none
Optimal	zucchini	none

Fruits

Poor	apple	B & E
MYF	apple juice	C & F
Poor	apple sauce (no sugar added)	B & E
Poor	apricots	B & E
Great	avocado	A
Risky	banana	C & E
Poor	blackberries	B & E
Poor	blueberries	B & E

Poor	cantaloupe	B & E
Poor	cherries	B & E
Poor	cranberries	B & E
Poor	dates	B & E
Poor	fig bar	B & E
MYF	fruit juice	C & F
Poor	grapefruit	B & E
Poor	grapes	B & E
Poor	honeydew melon	B & E
Poor	kiwi	B & E
Poor	mango	B & E
Poor	nectarine	B & E
Poor	orange	B & E
Poor	peach	B & E
Poor	pear	B & E
Poor	pineapple	B & E
Poor	plums	B & E
Poor	prunes	B & E
Poor	raisins	B & E
Poor	raspberries	B & E
Poor	strawberries	B & E
Poor	tangerine	B & E
Poor	watermelon	B & E

Carbohydrates

MYF	bagel	C & E
Good	beans, baked (vegetarian)	A & D
Good	beans, garbanzo	A & D
Risky	biscuits	C & E
Risky	blue corn chips	C & E

Risky	bread sticks	C & E
Risky	whole-wheat bread	C & E
Risky	hot dog or hamburger bun	C & E
Risky	cereal, Cheerios	C & E
Risky	clam chowder	C & E
MYF	cookies, fat free	C & F
Risky	corn	C & E
Risky	cornbread	C & E
Risky	corn on the cob	C & E
Risky	crackers, graham	C & E
Risky	cream of wheat	C & E
Risky	dinner roll	C & E
Risky	granola, nonfat	C & E
Risky	macaroni	C & E
MYF	muffin, blueberry or bran	C & F
Risky	muffin, english	C & E
Risky	noodles, egg, no yolk	C & E
Risky	oatmeal, cooked	C & E
Risky	pasta	C & E
Risky	popcorn, air popped	C & E
Risky	potato, baked with skin	C & E
MYF	french fries	C & F
Risky	potato, sweet	C & E
Risky	pretzels, hard	C & E
Risky	rice cakes	C & E
Risky	rice	C & E
Risky	soup, fat free	C & E
Risky	tortilla, flour	C & E
	Protein	
Optimal	bass	none

Good	beans, black/pinto	A & D
Optimal	beef, flank steak	none
Optimal	beef, ground round	none
Optimal	beef, lean cut	none
Optimal	beef, lean ground	none
Optimal	beef, round steak	none
Optimal	canadian bacon	none
Optimal	carp	none
Optimal	catfish	none
Great	cheese, cheddar	A
Great	cheese, fat free	A
Great	cheese, grated parmesan	A
Great	cheese, monterey jack	A
Great	cheese, mozzarella, part skim	A
Great	cheese, ricotta, whole milk	A
Great	cheese, swiss	A
Optimal	chicken breast, baked	none
Optimal	chicken, dark meat, no skin	none
Optimal	clams	none
Optimal	cod	none
Optimal	cold cuts	none
Great	cottage cheese	A
Optimal	eggs	none
Optimal	egg whites	none
Optimal	flounder	none
Optimal	haddock	none
Optimal	halibut	none
Optimal	lamb	none
Risky	lentils, cooked	C & E
Poor	milk, low fat	B & E

Good	peanut butter	A & D
Optimal	salmon, fresh	none
Optimal	scallops	none
Optimal	shrimp	none
Optimal	sole	none
Poor	tofu	B & E
Optimal	tuna, water packed	none
Optimal	turkey breast	none
MYF	yogurt, flavored, low fat	C & F
Good	yogurt, plain greek	A & D

Condiments

Good	thousand-island dressing	A & D
Good	thousand-island dressing, fat free	A & D
Good	blue-cheese dressing	A & D
Good	blue-cheese dressing, fat free	A & D
Good	butter	A & D
Great	cream cheese, Healthy Choice	A
Great	creamy italian dressing, no oil	A
Great	mayonnaise	A
Great	sour cream, light	A
Good	french dressing	A & D
Good	italian dressing	A & D
Good	margarine	A & D
Optimal	mustard	none
Good	ranch dressing, nonfat	A & D

Extra Credit Information.....

Why You Might Not Be Losing Weight

Healthy eating and weight loss go hand in hand for the most part. A diet filled with natural, whole foods is usually the best choice for people trying to lose weight, get healthier, or increase their performance in a sport. However, there are some exceptions to this rule. One of the most popular food choices for people looking to clean up their diet is fruit. If your immediate goal is just to lose weight, fruit can be detrimental to this process.

As most people know, fruit contains high levels of fructose (sugar). Fructose is absorbed quickly and spikes the fat-storage hormone insulin. If you are continuously pumping your body full of sugars like the ones found in fruit, your body will just be burning that for energy instead of the fat stored on your body, making it very difficult to lose weight. So although fruit offers a number of health benefits (antioxidants, vitamins, and minerals just to name a few), being overweight can trump most of them, making the risks outweigh the benefits.

If you are prioritizing and losing weight is your main goal, it is in your best interest to lower or eliminate your fruit consumption for a period of time. You can still get vital nutrients by replacing fruit with things like vegetables and nuts. If you do want to eat fruit make sure to do the proper level exercise first! Once you have improved your insulin sensitivity by following the *Do This, Eat That* plan consistently, your body will be able to better handle sugars such as the ones found in fruit, and they will have a more positive effect on your body composition.

Extra Credit Information.....

Stop the "Healthy Snacking"

When you open a magazine, or see an interview on TV by most "professionals" on how to eat healthier and lose weight, you most likely will hear them start with the phrase, "eat six to eight small meals per day." Now eating six to eight "small" meals per day can be conducive to better health if done correctly, but it will most likely prove to be detrimental to an individual's weight loss goals. Eating six to eight meals a day is a great way to keep blood sugar and insulin levels high. When you combine with the right macronutrient breakdown of food and training, it can really help pack on the mass. The trouble with this is the majority of the individuals getting this information are not looking to pile on the mass, but rather LOSE WEIGHT. If your goal is to lose weight, it is in your benefit to eat 2-3 larger meals of the correct macronutrient breakdown. First off this will keep your blood sugar spikes down, which will make your body more apt to burn fat. Secondly, eating a larger meal of the proper macronutrient breakdown, and actually getting FULL will make you feel less hungry throughout the day, along with controlling carb cravings. If you wait until you are actually hungry, that salmon and broccoli is going to taste like the best thing ever. If you have been eating small meals throughout the day, you are not going to be that hungry come meal time and you are much more apt to grab for the bread, or slice of pizza.

CHAPTER 5: MOVING FORWARD

The Right Way To Cut Calories

This is a plan that gives you all of the basics to achieve most weight loss, body composition, and fitness goals. Once you have followed this plan for a period of time, and have achieved some of your goals, this plan can be easily added or combined to a more specific plan with specific goals.

This plan is not centered on caloric intake, because caloric intake should be modified only when the body is functioning at an optimal level. This will ensure that when calories are reduced, fat is the primary energy source being burned. Following the *Do This, Eat That* Plan will do just this.

If your goal is to get down to that final cut for a wedding or photo-shoot, then is the time to start looking at your caloric intake. Once you have consistently followed this plan, and have practiced it for at least a month with no mistakes you can now start looking at your caloric intake. To do this, follow the amount of calories you are eating daily for about a week. When you are at a plateau (weight not going up or down), subtract two-hundred and fifty calories from your daily total. If your weight begins to reduce, then continue at that calorie total until you reach another plateau, at which point you will have to re-evaluate. If subtracting two hundred and fifty calories is not enough, then reduce weekly in two-hundred and fifty calorie increments until you reach a deficit and lose weight for the week. There are 3500 calories in a pound, so once your body is functioning optimally, a reduction of 250 calories a day comes out to be about a half pound loss per week, or two pounds per month. This may not seem like a lot, but because your body is functioning efficiently, this will be almost a one-hundred percent body fat lost. Also, losing weight in this manner, slowly and consistently, will allow for the highest percentage of body fat lost compared to muscle.

It is important to note that a restricted calorie diet is not advised for long periods of time. If fact, you will achieve better progress by having periods of time in which you are eating more calories per day. As long as you are fol-lowing the correct macronutrient breakdown as given to you in this plan, eating more calories for periods of time will actually benefit your metabolism in the long run. Simply put, make sure that the majority of your diet cen-ters around the plan outlined in this book, and utilize the proper way to cut calories for short term goals a couple times a year.

Your Basic Road Map to Training

This plan also focuses on giving you the basis for an all-inclusive training protocol. These basics are needed for any advanced fitness goals. Any individual regard-less of ability should learn the basics of all the exercises outlined in the *Do This* section of this book. These are also exercises that you should look to improve upon, and get stronger at in the long run. Improving your performance in these exercises both with the *Do This, Eat That* plan along with a regimen outside of the gym will allow for maximum success for the long run. Here is the basic outline for designing a training regimen for yourself involving the main exercise fundamentals outlined in this book.

If your goal is to also make progress in the gym, then follow this basic outline for putting together a program.

Start with an all-inclusive warm-up consisting of soft-tissue work, stretching, mobility work, and activation exercises. This will take different amounts of time depending on your limitations. Limitations can be anything from being sore and tight from your last session to trying to rehab an injury. In warming up you should gain a better understanding of your body and reach a level of preparedness that will allow you to get the best out of yourself each training session.

Your first lift should be a major compound lift, such as any variation of squatting, deadlifting, or pressing. Depending on your level, this can be anything from a modified push-up to a max-effort squat. No matter the movement, the whole idea of doing this first is to get stronger at that exercise. This is an instance where you are training the movement, not the muscles. The sole purpose for this movement is to hit a record for your-self on the exercise (basically meaning doing something you have never done before). Don't worry about muscle fatigue or trying to get a pump; just make sure you get stronger each week by increasing workload. You can increase workload three primary ways. The first way is to simply lift more weight than you have done before. Second you can lift a specific weight for more reps, or complete the same amount of work in less time. Lastly you can lift a weight faster, or with a higher rate of acceleration.

After your main lift, you should pick accessory work that hits your weaknesses. Between your warm-up and doing your main lift, you should gain a pretty good understand-ing of where your weaknesses are. Choose exercises that will hit these weaknesses. Doing this will help your prog-ress and lower your risk of injury.

Once you have completed your warm-up, main lift, and accessory work, now you can get into you specializations. If your goal is weight loss, then do some conditioning and cardio. If you are trying to pack on muscle, do some finishing sets to really overload the muscle and create a positive adaption.

Follow this basic roadmap to training, and you will be able to successfully design a training plan to accompany the *Do This, Eat That* plan, and work towards achieving even more specialized goals in fitness.

Extra Credit Information.....

2 Keys to Consistency

Here are some simple ways to help maintain consistency:

1. Focus on your main goals. If you have limited time, cut down excess parts of your program and still knock out the main stuff. Sometimes five to ten minutes of training can still keep you moving in the right direction.

2. Schedule time off from training that is part of your program. Not only is planning rest and recovery a pivotal component of making progress, it will also give you slots of times to make appointments and to take care of issues that occur outside of training.

CONCLUSION

This book was created specifically to teach you the right way to eat in order to change your body composition for the better. The *Do This, Eat That* program will turn you into a fat-burning, lean-mass-adding machine. This program alone will continuously improve your body composition and build a basic level of fitness that will give you a base for moving on to any fitness/performance goals you have. It is also designed to be a great addition to any training program. This book is not going to turn you into a high-level athlete, but it will give you the base to begin a training program that will take you in that direction. And if you are already a high-level athlete looking to clean up your diet, then you can implement these ideals within your current regimen.

There is no way around it: body re-composition takes a conscious effort to do things right. The high-carbohydrate, processed-food culture we live in today, along with increasingly more sedentary lifestyles, leaves the average person with a high body-fat percentage and a low amount of lean mass. Thanks to this culture, and the loads of poor information out there, this means that what is "comfortable" to the average person is a lifestyle that leads them to get progressively weaker and fatter. Being fat is the new norm, so if you want to be different, it takes doing things differently than the average person in today's world.

Changing things at first might feel a little uncomfortable, but soon your body will develop a new, more-positive habit of doing things right. It is important to remember that the principles of this plan adhere to the way in which our bodies are designed to function. If you are unhappy with how your body looks, or how it functions, it takes doing things differently to change that. You are not going to change by doing the same things that got you to that point to begin with.

All too often, decreased function and increased body fat percentage are attributed to age, but the truth is that for the most part we simply do it to ourselves. Age is one small piece of the puzzle that can be overcome by proper diet and training. This book has outlined a plan that can get each and every person who acts on it on the path to complete control over his or her body's composition.

This goes way beyond some numbers on the scale. Simply eating fewer calories overall might get you to drop some weight, but what weight is it? If you are eating a diet high in simple carbohydrates and low in protein and healthy fat, chances are you are dropping more muscle than fat. This can hurt you in a couple ways. First, losing weight in the form of muscle while maintaining your body fat usually will not get you the physique you are looking for. We've all seen the person who has dropped a ton of weight but now looks like he or she has an extra blanket of flab. By contrast, the *Do This, Eat That* plan will have you dropping the right weight (fat) and building muscle, which will get you looking more like a fitness model and less like a Chinese Shar-Pei.

Secondly, for function, health, and longevity, lean mass is needed. The amount of lean mass we have and can hold onto is directly related to our quality and duration of life. The health benefits of having a high percentage of lean body mass are huge. A high lean muscle mass means a higher percentage of good cholesterol, decreased blood pressure, and improved triglycerides/blood sugar, just to name a few benefits. Maintaining muscle mass and function is the key to staying independent as we enter into our twilight years. With all of this combined with a tighter body, why would anybody want to drop weight in the form of muscle?

This book lays out the groundwork for you to follow this science correctly and start getting the body you want today. You can find much more information about training and nutrition referenced in the index at the end of the book. Go to www.campotrained.com or www.riverwalkac.com to read new articles and blogs that will keep you updated and motivated, with the most amount of information possible. The key to overcoming the culture we live in is education!

Extra Credit Information.....

The Fountain of Youth

Through many interactions with people over the years in both personal training and physical therapy, people of all ages find it necessary to express how old they are and how they can't do the things like they used to. The interesting thing is that you hear the "it's tough getting old" comment from people anywhere from the age of twenty- five to one-hundred.

The truth is that age itself has very little to do with it. At some point people decide they are old and start limiting what they can do, using age as an excuse. For the most part, your body only ages if you let it. There is a law that speaks to this concept. According to Wolff's Law, (a theory developed by the anatomist and surgeon Julius Wolff,) the body responds to the demands placed on it. Stop placing demands on your body, and it will start withering away. Continue to put increasing demands on your body, and it will continue to grow and adapt.

Everybody is trying to find the fountain of youth. The nasty reality is that without proper care, our bodies literally deteriorate as we get older. This does not need to happen, and through a proper training program, such as *Do This, Eat That* you can reverse or slow down much of this aging process.

Many people are affected by osteoporosis as they get older. One of the main reasons this problem is such an epidemic is due to the lack of impact we place on our bones. As we get older and participate in less impactful activities, the body responds by breaking down bone (because the body thinks it is not needed) to ship calcium, amongst other things, out to be used in the rest of the body. By simply placing a bar on your back or participating in training that places impact on your bones, you can prevent this from happening in the first place. Even if you are already suffering from some level of osteoporosis, training can help build new bone density no matter what your age is.

Hormones are a strong driving force in the body. Decreasing levels of testosterone, for example, as we get older can lead to a handful of problems, including difficulty losing weight and adding lean muscle. Choosing high-intensity exercises such as back squats and performing them correctly can actually help boost testosterone levels, along with other hormones such as natural human growth hormone production.

As we get older, without a correct training regimen we build many muscle imbalances that inhibit our mobility and can cause all kinds of pain and disablement. Unfortunately, many of these issues in today's world are masked with pain pills and immobility. The only way to truly fix these problems is to locate and train the physical and chemical imbalances in the body. If you allow yourself to become more and more inactive as you get older, you will be speeding up the aging process. Through proper training you can address many of these issues to increase quality of life, and thus find the true fountain of youth.

APPENDIX

Correct Posture When Performing Exercises

Although each exercise has its own particular form, there are some basic principles regarding posture that you should focus on when performing most movements.

1. Arch the thoracic area of your back by squeezing your shoulder blades together (make believe you are putting your shoulder blades in your back pocket). Stick your chest out (make believe a string is pulling your chest toward the ceiling).
2. Brace your posture by taking in a big bellyful of air right before performing the movement, while staying as tight as possible. This will best activate your core and stabilize your balance and posture. This will also help to ensure no wasted movements. Top-level athletes make their performance seem effortless. This is a result of no wasted movements.
3. Focus your eyes on a point, and do not move them. Your body follows your eyes, so this will also help you to not make any wasted movement, and instead pay more attention to the exercise form. *Do not* close your eyes, as this will take away from your balance, and you will not be able to perform the exercise to your full capacity.

Flexibility Versus Stability

Joint mobilization is an important ingredient to any training program. However, many people confuse the difference between mobility and flexibility. Joint mobility is the ability to move a joint through its full range of motion. Joint mobility requires *stability* and *strength* of the joint in order to move properly and without injury.

Flexibility does not require strength. Instead, it is the ability to extend or flex a joint through its intended full range of motion. This pertains to the length of the tissue itself. When stretching for flexibility, the goal is to lengthen the tissue so that the joint can move freely through a range of motion with less restriction. Many people focus on flexibility stretching. While this will help to limit restrictions due to tightness of tissue, it does not do a great job of preparing your body to move quickly and efficiently.

Mobilizing a joint can help to distract the joint and oppose the normal accumulated compression that is constantly placed on the joint. Joint mobility work can also help to circulate synovial fluid and provide nutrients to the joint. This is a key component because the primary way a joint is nourished is through compression/distraction, and the circulation of synovial fluid. Without this the joint begins to lose its health. It is important to remember to take into consideration individual needs.

Depending on where the restriction or weakness is, the proper combination of both mobility and flexibility can help to best prepare the body for effective movement. It is important to understand that different joints have different needs. In a typically abled individual, the primary needs of the joints are as follows:

- Ankle - mobility (particularly sagittal (front to back))
- Knee - stability
- Hip - mobility (multiplanar, all directions)
- Lumbar (low back) - stability
- Thoracic (mid-back) - mobility
- Gleno-humeral (shoulder) - stability

Joints functioning correctly allow for optimal movement. While this is important for athletes and lifters trying to lift maximal weight, it can also help an individual see the need for specific training if one of these joints is lacking in either mobility or stability. Though there are always special cases, in large part injuries will occur if there is hypermobility in the joints that need stability such as the knee, lumbar spine, and glenohumeral joint. In contrast, injury often occurs when there is a lack of mobility (hypomobility) in joints like the ankle, hip, and thoracic spine.

Proper Shoulder Function

The "shoulder" as it is thought of is actually comprised of a number of joints and muscles other than just the gleno-humeral joint and muscles of the rotator cuff. You don't have to understand an in-depth analysis of all the components of the shoulder, but there are a couple key aspects that can ensure your shoulder is functioning optimally, and can prevent injury.

Although there are thousands of possible causes of shoulder pain and dysfunction, the most frequently treated injury in therapy is rotator cuff tendonitis. When thinking of shoulder function, one should begin proximally at scapular ("shoulder blades") function. Many times individuals will focus purely on the retraction and protraction of the scapula. Although someone might have what appears to be good scapular mobility through retraction and protraction, if the scapula is not rotating properly it could start a cycle of dysfunction and pain distally down the chain into the shoulder and down the arm. For most individuals, pulling and pressing movements require the scapula to downwardly rotate during the retraction phase, and upwardly rotate during the protraction phase. Being able to demonstrate this movement pattern will allow not only for proper force translation, but also will properly stabilize the scapula which will allow for optimal motor unit recruitment and inter/intra-muscular coordination. Long story short, this equals bigger lifts with a lower chance of injury. If the scapula is not rotating properly it can lead to multiple dysfunctional patterns that can be seen through a movement assessment. It is important to remember that learning a proper movement pattern first involves motor learning planning through the Central Nervous System. This means plenty of frequency in practicing this pattern is needed in order to develop the proper motor plan.

The best way to describe downward and upward rotation of the scapula during retraction and protraction is to use your hands. Stick your hands straight out in front of you like you are about to grab two doorknobs. Pull your hands in towards your chest, and as you do this rotate your hands so that your thumbs go up and your pinkies goes down (Pinkies are mimicking acromion.) This is replicating retraction with downward rotation (your hands being the scapula.) As you press your hands back out so they are straight out in front of you, rotate your hands back so that your pinkies go up, and your thumbs turn down. This is mimicking protraction with upward rotation. Get the movement pattern down, and begin practicing it as often as possible when you are doing pulling and pressing movements to master proper shoulder function!

Proper Push-Ups

Push-ups are an exercise that should be a part of everyone's training in one way or another. If you are not able to do a full push-up, then it is important to be developing the all-around strength and intra-muscular coordination that you need to be able to do this important exercise. As a strength athlete, push-ups will better teach you how to turn a bench press into a closed-chain movement, thus maximizing your strength potential. Someone looking to add muscle to their physique can add high-frequency push-ups into their regimen to help to build some pretty impressive arms, back, and chest. As someone looking for general fitness and health, push-ups will give you a better base of total body strength and help to build a strong core and stable joints.

There are many different variations of push-ups that can be trained, but for the purpose of learning the basics, the traditional push-up will be the focus of this section.

Stability initially needs to be present in order to perform a "full" push-up. A "full" push-up is being able to keep your body in correct posture and move through the full range of motion (arms locked to chest to ground, and back to arms locked) without breaking form. Perpendicular to the ground, the landmarks of your shoulders, fore-arms, and palms should be as close as possible to a straight line. Your back should be in normal curvature and remain in such throughout. For your back to be in proper curvature, you should be able to draw a straight line from the landmarks of your head to your shoulders to your butt. There might be slight variances among different people depending on the length of their levers. However, your goal should be as close to a straight line as possible with the landmarks mentioned. No matter what width of stance or grip, you should try to maintain this posture.

The following will discuss the mechanics of a proper pushup down the chain of movement.

Bio-mechanics of the push-up

Starting at the top, you should keep your head back and lead with your chest. When certain weaknesses or poor mechanics are present, many people will try to lead the movement with their head. This is improper; you should lead with your chest instead of your head. To better facilitate proper movement keep a neutral head, and pinch your shoulder blades together by retracting your shoulder blades (scapula). This will put you in position to lead with your chest. The scapula should also be in a position of downward rotation. To best facilitate this movement, while in the top, locked-out position before your descent to ground, you should downwardly rotate and retract the scapula (see also "Proper Shoulder Function.") This position will give you the most power in that all the muscles of your back will be able to stabilize the movement. As you descend, your elbows should bend at approximately forty-five degrees. When you begin coming up, near the top of your movement you should "spread the floor" to facilitate upward rotation of the scapula, and maximize optimal tricep function and lockout power.

The core can be generalized by including all of the muscles from the knees to the sternum. During the movement you should help stabilize the core by taking a big belly breath to build intra-abdominal pressure. Having a stable core is usually the biggest problem people have with being able to accomplish a push-up. Although many people possess the upper-body strength to push up their body weight, they are not able to stabilize their core throughout the movement.

Modifying push-ups is all about manipulating the job of the core. If a weakness is present, you will often see people break form by pushing their butt in the air or allowing their hips to sag to the floor. Again, you should try to maintain a straight line from the head to the shoulders to the butt. When your break out of this form due to a weak core, you translate the energy used and decrease your maximum strength potential. You should begin at a level in which you can maintain this posture throughout for the most part.

Depending on your level, you can start as easy as on a wall. You can challenge yourself further by moving down lower to a counter, table, or chair. The eventual goal is being able to get all the way to the ground. When you can successfully do at least one rep while maintaining proper posture, this should be considered your current strength level. Your stability level will be at least one level less challenging than your strength level. So this means you should perform a stability exercise such as isometric planks, which are a training tool for building the strength and stability necessary to do push-ups, at a level lower to the ground than your current strength level. For example, if you're current strength level only allows you to do push-ups on the wall; you should perform planks on a counter. For the planks, hold and stabilize the posture we have discussed at the top position for a period of time.

Some good schemes to use are three sets of thirty seconds or ten sets of ten seconds. As you get stronger, continue to move your way down toward the ground for push-ups while performing planks at one level closer to the ground than your push-ups.

Now, once you are able to successfully perform planks from the ground, maintaining proper posture for at least one set of thirty seconds, you can begin modified push-ups from the ground. The first modified position is actually starting with your body all the way on the floor. Instead of starting from lockout, or top-plank, position, start from the ground, push yourself up to your knees, and then lift your knees up into a plank. Once at the top, lower yourself under as much control as possible, maintaining proper posture until you are all the way on the ground. If you start off "flopping" on the floor, this is quite OK; just maintain control for as long as possible.

As you get stronger, you will be able to lower yourself with more and more control. Also as you get stronger, you will be able to spend less and less time on your knees on the up part of the push-up. Try to more quickly transition from knees to plank until you barely need your knees at all. Pretty soon you will be able to start from the top position and do a full push-up! Using this method will best train your core along with all your other upper-body muscles to best teach intra-muscular coordination and get you pounding out plenty of proper push-ups.

Another key point to remember is that this is a *training* process. Everybody will start at different parts of a training spectrum. It is not about where your start; however, it is about where you end up. It will take plenty of time and work, but anybody, at any level, can train to be able to do better push-ups. Once you are able to do full push-up, continue to challenge yourself by performing as many as you can continuously, or adding resistance with a bands or weights.

Squat Mechanics for the Beginner

Are squats right for you? Yes! If you can sit down and stand up, this means you can squat. Since you do this multiple times per day, it would be in your best interest to develop a proper motor plan for this movement. If you are not healthy or strong enough to stand up, then you must be put on a plan or program than works on properly progressing you to be able to perform this movement. The ability to get up and down has been shown to be directly correlated with our quality of life as we get older.

It doesn't matter who you are; squats can positively impact every aspect of your training. Whether you are trying to lose weight, pack on the muscle, or maintain your quality of life while performing daily functions through better fitness, improving your squat will be highly beneficial.

First let's identify what it meant by a "full squat." A full squat is being able to drop your hips so that the point of your hip (iliac crest) is below the knee. This usually results in the thighs being at least parallel to the ground. The reason that depth is important is because this is the proper depth that needs to be reached in order to successfully and properly be able to get up off the ground with proper form. A proper squat involves going to this depth with no prominent break in posture. Maintaining correct posture throughout the entire range of motion is the key for developing functional strength.

Bio-mechanics of the squat

Like most exercises, breathing is very important. Before each repetition or movement, you should focus on the coordination of proper breathing. Take a deep breath right before you perform the eccentric (for the squat this would be the downward movement) portion of the movement. Use the breath to create intra-abdominal pressure and brace your posture to facilitate proper mechanics.

Starting at the cervical spine, you should tuck your chin back into cervical retraction in order to facilitate proper mechanics down the chain of movement. This is very important because the rest of the body usually follows the head, and this can be a pivotal component of improving your squat.

The thoracic spine (upper back) posture should consist of the shoulder blades being squeezed together in order to stabilize the lumbar spine (lower back,) and keep your back in proper alignment. There should be no movement of the spine itself during a squat. Pinching your shoulder blades together and keeping your lats and core tight will maintain this.

Next, let's discuss the hips. This is where mobility should take place during the squat. Maintaining the proper curvature of the spine while you drive your hips back will allow you to descend properly. You want to open your hips up by pushing your legs apart (like you are trying to spread the floor) and sitting back while maintaining a stabile back. You should have your legs spaced apart a distance that allows you to open your hips up and sit back the best. This will allow you to properly engage your glutes, hamstrings, and quads to perform the movement. This will also get the muscles of your back to fire and maintain proper stability. Depending on your levers, pushing your butt back properly might result in leaning forward. This is fine as long as you maintain the proper curvature in the back, because leaning forward will just result in a hinge of the lower back/hip area and not place any additional stresses like shearing on the back. If you are tall and have very long levers, you will have to bend forward more than the average person in order to maintain proper form down the chain of movement. It is important for tall individuals to really focus on keeping their chests up (thoracic extension) in order to compensate for this.

Next down the chain of movement is the knee joint. Due to an inability to properly use the hips, a lot of people will translate too much mobility into the back and the knees. This is usually the cause of injury in association with the squatting movement. The idea is to keep your knees stabile with no excess movement that usually results in shearing forces on the knee. Shearing forces are forces that are improperly applied to joint, and can cause damaging wear and tear. Proper form will result in the force being applied to the muscles, not the joint, and will dramatically reduce the chance of injury over time. Proper movement at the knee joint basically means your knees should not protrude forward past your feet. If you are maintaining stability in your back and sitting back with your hips in order to achieve depth, there should be next to no movement with the knee itself other than a slight bend. The key is to never stop pushing your butt back and opening your hips up by "spreading the floor" (as discussed earlier). The second you stop pushing your butt back and opening your hips up, you will translate the energy into your knees, and your knees will protrude forward. The translation into the knee results in shearing forces that could potentially be damaging.

If you have perfectly healthy knees, this might not be as much of an issue and you probably can get away with some forward-protruding knees. It might even help you get better quad development and strength. However, if avoiding injury is your primary focus, you will want to work on driving those hips back, with little to no move-ment in the spine and knees. It is important to note that form doesn't always have to be perfect, and you must train the movement frequently to get better at it. Even though no one in the world has perfect squat form, your goal should still be to have the best possible form for yourself, while still training the movement consistently.

The tracking of the knees is very important as well. Your knees should track directly over your toes throughout the movement. If your knees track out (genu varum) or track in (genu valgum,) this will once again result into translation of energy into damaging shearing forces onto the knee.

Ankle mobility is an often-forgotten component of proper squat form. Similar to your hips, your ankles need to be actively mobile to facilitate proper function in the movement. While the hips need to be mobile in multiple directions, the ankles primarily need to be mobile anterior to posterior (sagittal.) If there is not enough ankle mobility in this plane, the energy will again usually translate into excess movement of your knees. Proper ankle mobility work might be necessary to help with proper squat form. Your feet should be spaced far enough apart in order to keep the heel of your foot on the ground. This is extremely important because the movement should be driven through the heels of the foot in order to maintain optimal movement up the chain. Typically, proper feet spacing is slightly wider than shoulder width, with the feet slightly pointed outward.

Everyone has a unique body structure that will in some way hinder "perfect" squat form. The key is to identify these weaknesses and continue to progress. Things like the stretching of tight hips and ankles, and stabilizing and strengthening the core will help. However, simply focusing on the correct form by training and getting stronger at the movement, along with developing an efficient motor plan, will help to correct many of the issues that are there initially. As you continue to get stronger, a lot of these problems, such as "tight hips," will start to dissipate. If the problems persist, then a specialization program should be instituted to fix them.

With the goal being to perform a full squat and then to increase added resistance, you must first reach full range of motion without compromising posture. Start at whatever depth you can get to with the proper form. To start, use a chair, table, or box to squat to because you will have a goal to reach every time. A good base rule to use for progression is that if you can perform five good bodyweight reps at a given height, you can move the box lower or use a smaller chair or table. There is a misconception that if you can't do something a hundred times, then you "can't" do it. Strength is what you can perform in one all-out effort. So even if you can only do three reps, your one-rep max will most likely be at a lower depth that what you used for the three reps. The key point here is that when training for strength, the reps need to be challenging in order to force a positive body adaption. Therefore, you should train ranges that are challenging. You are not going to get stronger by training a depth you can consistently and easily hit for twenty reps.

It is important to remember that even if you can only do an exercise for one good rep, you *can* do it.

Another good tool to help teach proper posture through a full range is "stripper squats." Stand in front of a pole or railing, and use it to balance as you sit back. This will help you see the correlation between depth, pushing your butt back, and your knees not protruding forward. This is a great tool for people with poor balance and/or ankle mobility. This exercise will help also increase range through mobility of the hips.

Once you can achieve full range with proper posture, you can add resistance/load. Different variations of squats involve a few new steps of posture in regard to holding additional weight, such as a bar, however all of these basics will continue to hold true.

Optimal Gait Most people have the ability to walk or run in some fashion. The idea is to become biomechanically sound in order to increase your current level (e.g., advancing from walking to running) and lower your risk of injury in the long term. You want mechanics that will allow for optimal intra-muscular coordination along with a good balance between agonist and antagonist (opposing) muscle groups. For optimal and efficient gait, opposing muscle groups are best used together in order to move in an energy-efficient manner, along with maintaining a balance of muscles in the body. For optimal and efficient gait, the gluteal muscles and hamstrings are quite possibly the most important muscles. Proper mechanics are facilitated through proper use of these muscles. The gluteal muscles and hamstrings should be concentrically used in "push off" or propulsion. These muscles are used eccentrically during swing to stabilize the terminal swing leg itself. Immediately before and during this stage of swing, the opposite leg is transitioning from the loading response and mid-stance to terminal stance. In this transition, the stance leg can concentrically activate in the hamstrings and gluteal muscles to "push off" and help propel the body. Right after mid-stance of the stance leg, active propulsion should be engaged by concentric contraction of the hamstrings and gluteal muscles. (Yessis Michael (2011) Explosive Running. Second Ed. Ultimate Athlete Concepts.)

To complete the movement, using optimum balance, the hip flexors (opposing muscle group to the glutes and hamstrings) should be used eccentrically to contract and stabilize the pelvis. In the swing leg, there is a concentric contraction of the hip flexors, and an eccentric contraction of the gluteal muscles and hamstrings to help stabilize the pelvis. There are many other things going on here to stabilize the pelvis (e.g., concentric contraction of gluteus medius during mid-stance of stance leg to stabilize pelvic drop); however, initially one should just focus on the balance of gluteus maximus/hamstrings and hip flexors in order to begin training an optimal gait pattern. Using the concentric contraction of the standing legs' glutes and hams while the hip flexors stabilize, along with using the concentric contraction of the hip flexors in the swing leg while the glutes and hams stabilize will allow for the best balance and force dispersion. (Tupa VV, Guesinov FA, Mironenko IN (1991) "Fatigue-Induced Changes in Sprinting Technique." Soviet Sports, Review 26.)

As we know, the body wants to be balanced, so if the body is trained to function this way, it will allow for optimal force production. Force production is directly related to stride length. The more force, the longer the stride length and the less strides that need to be taken. Fewer strides make for a more-efficient gait. Another very important point is that training for this optimal balance between muscles such as the hams/glutes and hip flexors will lower the chance of injury. If a muscular imbalance develops, such as stronger hip flexors/quads and weaker hams/gluts (such that might happen if proper "push off" is not used), risk of knee injury is increased. When agonist/antagonist muscles are not properly balanced, atypical translation (improper force applied to joints) can occur in surrounding joints, thus adding additional wear and tear on that joint.

Proper Lunges

Lunges and all of their variations are a great unilateral (single-leg) exercise that can serve a multitude of purposes when training. Lunges can be a great tool that helps tremendously with strength training, fat loss, conditioning, and all-around function. Most repetitive functional activities we do during a day such as going up and down stairs are single-leg movements.

In order to help prevent wear and tear on the body, it is in your best interest to learn how to do a basic single-leg movement, like lunges, correctly, in order to train the proper muscles that will help protect your joints in the long run. From a strength perspective, lunges help bring balance in the development of the body, which means that along with promoting strength gains you will build a better, more symmetrical physique. Once the movement is learned and performed correctly, lunges can also be done in certain intensities to help positively train the cardiovascular system. Utilizing the correct performance of lunges will strengthen you, help you build muscle, keep you injury-free, and allow you to train at a higher intensity, which is the long-term solution to proper fat loss.

The first reason people have trouble with single-leg movements such as lunges, is balance. When looking to improve balance, you must first learn proper breathing. Breathing correctly will get you "tight" and optimize your motor-unit recruitment in the muscles. Many people can help train and fix balance deficits through proper breathing. If you are breathing properly and getting optimum recruitment but are still having balance issues, then you should look into other areas such as ankle strength and vestibular testing.

Proper breathing consists of taking your time in between every rep, taking in a big breath of air, swallowing the air into your stomach, and holding it tight through the movement. The air should come out passively as you complete the movement. The idea is to repeat this for each rep and not hold your breath for too long or for too many reps. Along with the recruitment you are facilitating through this type of breathing, you are also getting the oxygen that you need to fuel each repetition.

Biomechanics of the Lunge

The basic walking lunge means that you are taking a step forward, dropping your back knee all the way to the ground, pushing through your front foot's heel, stabilizing through both legs, and pulling yourself up with your front leg to bring your back foot even with the front.

The first region we will discuss is that of the head, chest, and upper back. The head should be back in cervical retraction in order to facilitate proper posture. Shoulder blades must be squeezed together in order to stabilize the lumbar spine (lower back) and keep the back in proper alignment. There should be no movement of the spine itself (flexion/extension) during a lunge. Pinching shoulder blades together and staying tight will maintain this. To also help facilitate this movement, keep your eyes looking up and your head in cervical retraction. Stick your chest out ("chest high") to also help facilitate proper movement. Notice this is very similar the mechanics of the squat as discussed in "Squat Mechanics for the Beginner."

Take a long enough step so that your feet are far enough apart to bring your knee straight down to the ground. A common problem is that the step is not long enough, which means the person will shift his or her weight too far forward as he or she goes down to account for the shift in the center of gravity. This essentially means you are wasting your energy and making the movement less efficient. Also, training and learning these improper mechanics will most likely result in doing single-leg functional movements like stairs throughout the day incorrectly. This improper movement will wear down your joints over time and can cause a variety of health problems.

For proper alignment, make sure that when you step both feet are pointed forward. You may not be able to have both feet pointed completely forward depending on how you are built, imbalances, and your ability level. Just remember to keep them as straight forward as possible. Feet slightly pointed out is alright, as this will help you use your hips better. Just remember if your feet are pointed out, make sure to push your knees out also so that they continue to track over the feet throughout the movement. As you get stronger, many times some small postural issues will clear up as long as you are focusing on correcting them each time. So continue to train the movement at a high frequency to the best of your ability, but not every rep has to be perfect.

To review, take a big breath to keep your head, chest, and upper back in proper alignment, and take a long enough step in which the back knee goes into a straight line right down to the ground.

The next region is the hips, knees, and ankles. Make sure you bring your knee all the way to the ground, but do not just drop it. It should be brought down under control and lightly tap the ground. The majority of your weight should be the heel of the front foot, and you should keep your shoulder in alignment with your hips throughout the movement. Leaning too far forward or back will again translate and waste energy. To come up, drive that front heel through the floor in order to pull your back foot up so that it is even with the front foot. Stand tall with the same good posture at the top of each rep. Once you complete the lunge on one side, take another big breath and step with the other foot to repeat.

What do you do if you cannot perform a full lunge yet? Similar to other exercises (refer to "Proper Squat Mechanics for the Beginner," Pull-up Progressions" and "Proper Push-Ups"); there is a series of progressions you can use to build the strength necessary to be able to eventually do a lunge. The idea is to always remember the key points discussed at the beginning of this section, and to maintain that form through the modifications. If the form breaks down doing just one rep at a given level, you should train at the level right before that one until you are able to move on to the next level.

To begin the lunge progression, as you perform the lunge, only bring your knee down to a level where you can maintain form. This can be anything from only dropping down an inch to going all the way to the floor. Again, you should start at one level before form breaks down. So, for example, if you can successfully bring your knee down 50 percent to the floor and maintain proper form for three solid reps on each side, this is a good place to start. Eventually as you continuously train the movement, you may be able to drop the knee 60 percent of the way to the floor and perform the same amount of quality reps. Progression is the key to making strength gains, and this is a simple way to judge strength progression of lunges.

If you have access to a variety of different box-step heights, you can use those for reps as well. Step with one foot on either side of the box, with both feet pointing forward, and drop your knee so that it touches the box or step. As you get stronger, you can use a lower step or box. This can be a great way to train and progress lunges because it gives you a consistent level to go to each time. Once you become proficient at a full bodyweight lunge, you can add resistance by holding weights.

Progressing Pull-ups

Any variations of pull-ups are a great exercise for achieving almost any fitness goal. The problem is that your
standard pull-up is much more challenging for the typical
individual than other bodyweight exercises such as push-
ups, squats, lunges ect... The good news is that there
are many variations of pull-ups that you can use to train
your current level. The key is to identify your level, train
it, and then progress to the next level over time. The
following will teach you to do just this.

Traditionally when someone refers to a pull-up, they
are referring to a prone (palms facing away from face)
grip. For the typical individual a chin-up, which is a supine
(palms facing towards face) grip, is usually slightly eas-
ier. There is also a neutral grip chin-up which is about
halfway between the two, with the thumbs facing towards
the face. For the purpose of discussing form and progression, grip width (how far the hands are apart) is not
that important, so just always start with about a shoulder
width grip or whatever is most comfortable. Just note
that you can train many different grip widths to help hit
the muscles just a little differently.

The variations and progressions of pull-ups/chin-ups are
listed in order from least to most challenging.

There are a few form and technique practices you should implement on all of these. Always stay as tight as possible as to facilitate as much motor unit recruitment as possible. Squeeze the bar, your lats, and your glutes as much as possible. Take a big breath, and push it into your stomach to brace your core right before the lift.

1.) The first method to modify is the angle of the body. Pull-ups/Chin-ups are a vertical pulling motion, which due to how forces are applied is the most challenging in regards to an individual's bodyweight. An inverted row is a great place to start because it is a horizontal pulling motion, in which more of the bodyweight can be displaced. With a bar about 3 feet off the floor, start with a supine grip. Pull your bodyweight up and try to touch your chest to the bar. If you still cannot pull your full bodyweight up, keep your feet flat on the floor, and use your hips and posterior chain to help lift your bodyweight up. If this is still too challenging, sit more upright, and pull just your upper body to the bar, leaving the lower body sitting on the floor. As you get stronger, bring your feet further away from your body and try to just use your upper body to lift your chest to the bar. As you progress try a prone grip.

2.) Once you become comfortable with the inverted row, seated pull-ups/chin-ups are the next variation. For this movement you will need an adjustable bar (ex. Smith Machine.) Set the bar up to about chest height. Place a chair underneath the bar. Grab the bar and pull your weight up. Use your legs to help you lift your bodyweight up, and lift your chest to the bar. The key is to only use as much legs as you need, and pull as much as possible to get your bodyweight up to the bar. As you progress and get stronger use less and less legs. Once like you feel like you can lift the majority of your weight with no leg assistance you can move to the next level.

3.) The next level is assisted pull-ups. There is a couple ways you can perform this exercise. Many gyms have an assisted pull-up machine that has a platform you can stand on to reduce the amount of your bodyweight you are lifting. This is a great tool to use, and allows you to progress simply by reducing the amount of assistance the machine is giving you. If you do not have access to one of these machines you can also use bands. Anchor the band to the bar so that there is a loop that hangs down. You can insert your knee into the loop, and the band will provide you some assistance depending on the strength of the band. As you get stronger simply reduce the strength of the band that is assisting you. A pivotal component of what will get you to the next level is your core. Even though you are being assisted by a machine or bands, make sure to get a nice big breath and engage your entire core as much as possible. If you are swinging while performing the movement, you are still not utilizing your core. If the core is weak, make sure to really focus on your breathing and keeping everything tight to help and progress you to the next level. Once you can perform pull-ups comfortably at the least amount of assistance that you have at your disposal, it is time for the next level.

4.) Now it's time to truly start mastering you bodyweight. Jumping and eccentric pull-ups are great way to do just this. For these you might need to put a step or box under the pull-up bar so you can reach and grab the bar from standing. Start with jumping pull-ups. Simply jump as much as you need to get your chin over the bar. Again, as you progress use only as much "jump" as you need to get your chin over the bar. If this is too challenging, use a higher step or box. For eccentric pull-ups, start with your chin above the bar by standing on a high enough box, and then lower yourself down under control until you are completely hanging with outstretched arms. Stand back up on the box and repeat the eccentric movement until you can no longer control your bodyweight. Remember to breathe and brace your core to try and prevent excessive swinging. It is also important to note that the reps do not have to be perfect, challenge yourself to get your body to progress! Once you have successfully performed both jumping and eccentric pull-ups, try to combine them by doing a jumping pull-up, and then controlling yourself all the way down. Also remember to train supine, neutral and prone grips as you progress and get stronger.

5.) Once you can pull yourself up to the bar with no jump you are able to do full pull-ups or chin-ups! Continue working to solidify your form. Once you can perform a few reps in a row try to challenge yourself further by adding resistance. Again, the reps don't have to be perfect, the most important thing as that you continue to challenge yourself through the overload principle. The overload principle says that as you keep increasing the demands, your body will adapt to account for the new demands placed on it.

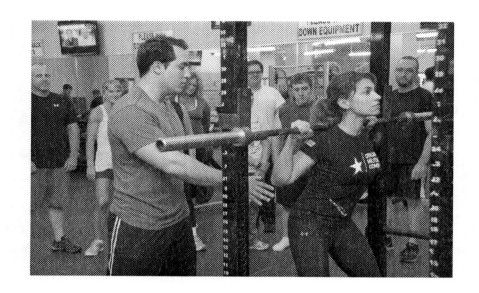

About the Authors

Anthony Campo is a licensed Physical Therapist Assistant, and is a member of the Phi Theta Kappa International Honor Society. He is also a Certified Personal Trainer through the National Exercise & Sports Trainers Association (NESTA,) and Certified Nutritional Consultant through Penn Foster University. Anthony has a wealth of hands on knowledge and has been actively practicing in the field since 2008. He specializes in strength and conditioning, corrective flexibility and mobility, and diet and meal planning. He has trained/treated a large variety of clientele, helping them to achieve a wide spectrum of goals. His experience ranges from pediatrics to geriatrics, young athletes to elite level athletes, and disabled individuals to persons with special needs. Learn more about Anthony Campo at www.CampoTrained.com.

Kristina Martemucci lives in upstate New York where she works as the General Manager of an athletic club and where she conducts her personal training business, Perfect Fit.   After receiving her Master's degree in Education from Pepperdine University and teaching for a number of years, she went on to pursue her personal training certification through the National Academy of Sports Medicine and started her own business in 2007.   Shortly thereafter Kristina received her Specialist in Fitness Nutrition Certification from the International Sports Sciences Association.   In combination with her qualifications and experience she has been able to work with, reach, and change the lives of many people of all fitness and health backgrounds.   Learn more about Kristina Martemucci at www.kmdperfectfittraining.com